# HANDBOOK OF
# SPINAL CORD MEDICINE

# Handbook of Spinal Cord Medicine

**DAVID C. BURKE**, M.B., B.S., D.P.R.M.,
*Medical Director, Spinal Injuries Unit, Austin Hospital, Heidelberg, Victoria, Australia*

**D. DUNCAN MURRAY**, M.D., F.R.C.P.(C.),
*Assistant Medical Director (Acting), Spinal Injuries Centre, and Lecturer in Rehabilitation Medicine, Dalhousie University, Canada*

**MACMILLAN**

First published 1975
Reprinted 1984, 1986

Published by
MACMILLAN EDUCATION LTD
Houndmills, Basingstoke, Hampshire RG21 2XS
and London
Companies and representatives
throughout the world

Printed in Hong Kong

ISBN 0-333-18711-3

# PREFACE

This handbook is designed as a pocket companion for new doctors working in a Spinal Unit or Rehabilitation Department. It serves as an introductory text for the young resident or house doctor who has had no previous experience with the specialised problems of the spinal paralytic, providing a brief overview of the whole subject. A sample of more detailed texts are referred to in the Bibliography for further reading.

The handbook should also quickly gain acceptance amongst medical students as it provides a concise source of information about a specialised topic which is not found in standard student texts. It will also have a useful place in the orientation of new nursing staff, physiotherapists, occupational therapists and other paramedical staff who are called upon to treat paraplegics and tetraplegics. As such, it should also have a useful place in schools of nursing, physiotherapy, etc.

Physicians treating patients with spinal cord injuries will quickly realise the value of this pocket handbook when new staff of all disciplines commence work in their Centres, just as the authors have in their respective Units in Melbourne and Halifax.

D.C.B.
D.D.M.

# CONTENTS

# FUNCTIONAL ANATOMY OF THE SPINAL COLUMN

## General Description

The vertebral column is classically divided into various levels: the 7 cervical vertebrae, 12 thoracic, 5 lumbar, 5 sacral and 4 coccygeal.

The articulating parts of these vertebrae are the vertebral bodies which are separated by invertebral discs, and the posterior facet joints of the pedicles. The former tend to be the weight-bearing joints, and the latter function as sliding and gliding joints.

Within the vertebral column, the spinal cord is protected ventrally by the posterior aspect of the vertebral body, dorsally by the bony laminae, and laterally by the pedicles. As well as the posterior articulating surfaces, each pedicle has superior and inferior grooves which form the invertebral foramina through which the spinal nerves pass.

Important ligamentous structures include the anterior and posterior longitudinal ligaments, both of which have intimate attachment to the vertebral bodies and disc spaces. There is a tough posterior interspinous ligament joining the dorsal aspects of the spinous processes. The thick, short ligamentum flavum covers the interlaminar spaces. The posterior articulating facets have joint capsules. All these ligaments contribute to the stability of the vertebral column.

Dentate ligaments help to fix the spinal cord in a central position in the canal, but it is still able to move as much as 9 mm in an anterior–posterior direction.

## Cervical Vertebrae

The convex occipital condyles articulate with the first cervical vertebra, or atlas. The movement of this occipito-atlantal joint is limited in flexion and extension. Between the atlas and axis (C2) there is an unusual joint. The posterior surface of the anterior arch of C1 has a facet which is in contact with the protruding odontoid process of C2. There is a strong transverse ligament joining the two lateral masses of the atlas and passing posteriorly to the odontoid. Other major ligaments attach the odontoid to the inner aspect of the occipital condyles and anterior margin of the foramen magnum. This arrangement allows rotation. Some flexion and extension is also allowed. The anterior arch of C1 remains 1 mm from the odontoid in flexion and extension. If there is widening of this space greater than 3 mm one suspects damage to the transverse ligament of the atlas.

The remainder of the cervical vertebrae are similar in appearance. The articular processes are found at the junction of the pedicles and laminae. The inferior facets face downward and forward, and glide on the superior facet of the vertebrae below. There are small neurocentral joints located laterally between the cervical vertebral bodies. The vertebral artery runs in the foramen transversarium of the transverse processes of C2–C6.

The average sagittal diameter of the cervical vertebral canal is 18 mm. Maximal movement of the cervical spine takes place at C5–C6.

Degenerative arthritic changes in this area may encroach upon the narrow bony canal. As the cervical cord is at its maximum width at this level, there is a great risk of neurological damage secondary to injury.

### Thoracic and Lumbar Vertebrae

In the thoracic spine the vertebrae are similar, and so constructed that there is only a limited range of movement. This consists of a little flexion and extension and minimal rotation. This is explained by the direction of the articular facets. The direction of the superior facets is posterio-lateral and the inferior facets face anterio-medial. The transverse processes articulate with the ribs in the thoracic spine, which further restricts motion.

In the lumbar spine, again the vertebrae are similar, but there is a greater provision for flexion, and to a lesser degree, extension. The plane of the articular facets changes from medial-lateral to anterior-posterior as one proceeds from L1–L5.

The spinal cord ends opposite the L1–L2 vertebral body level in the adult. Below this the elements of the cauda equina are within the vertebral canal of the lumbar spine. The mobility of the cauda equina roots in the large canal provides a safety factor not found in the cervical or thoracic levels.

## Arterial Supply of the Spinal Cord

Each vertebral artery contributes a branch at the brainstem to form a single anterior spinal artery. This runs the length of the cord lying over the median fissure. It tapers as it runs caudally in the thoracic cord.

Each vertebral artery also contributes to a posterior spinal artery on the same side. As they progress distally, they form longitudinal plexiform channels.

The superior portion of the anterior spinal artery is re-inforced by radicular arteries around the C3 level. These enter through the intervertebral foramina. The most constant radicular artery is around C6–C7.

There are few radicular arteries supplying the upper thoracic cord. A large radicular artery, the great spinal artery, enters between the T9–L3 level. This may be responsible for between a quarter and a half of the blood supply of the cord below this level.

At intervals of about 2 mm the anterior spinal artery gives off central branches which, in turn, branch peripherally and centrally.

It is felt that the anterior spinal artery supplies all the cord with the exception of the posterior columns and posterior horns which are supplied by the posterior spinal arteries. Some feel that the anterior spinal artery is the main source of blood supply to the posterior arteries below the upper thoracic level.

The arterial system of the cord does not have extensive collateral circulation and relies on the extraspinal radicular arterial sources. Any interruption of these can produce serious neurological damage.

## SECTION 2

# FUNCTIONAL ANATOMY OF THE SPINAL CORD

### General Description

There is an enlargement in the lower cervical spinal cord giving rise to the brachial plexus. Another enlargement is seen in the segments from where the lumbo-sacral plexus arises.

In cross-section the cord reveals the grey central cord surrounded by white matter. The butterfly-shaped grey matter is composed of cell bodies of the neurons with their branching dendritic processes. It owes its colour to the paucity of medullated fibres.

Its dorsal horn cells receive fibres from the dorsal roots and give rise to fibres ascending in the spinothalamic and spinocerebellar tracts. Terminal axons of visceral afferents also travel in this portion of the spinal cord.

The intermediate column of grey matter is present only in the thoracic, lumbar and sacral portions of the cord. In the thoracic and lumbar cord it contains the cells of origin for the preganglionic fibres of the sympathetic nervous system. The sacral intermediate column contains the para-sympathetic pathways, and fibres pass out in corresponding ventral roots to end on post-ganglionic neurons near the organ supplied.

The ventral horn contains large multipolar neurons characteristic of efferent cells. The axons emerge to enter the ventral roots.

4

The white matter contains glistening sheaths of longitudinally-running medullated fibres. The tracts usually ascend or descend vertically, but may be tangential or horizontal in passing through the grey matter to the opposite side. Ascending paths are sensory: descending paths are motor.

## Ascending Tracts

The *lateral spinothalamic* tract carries pain and temperature fibres. They enter through the posterior roots and ascend in the tracts of Lissauer for a few segments before terminating on second-order neurons in the grey matter of the dorsal horn. Fibres from these neurons cross the anterior commissure, pass to the opposite lateral column and form the lateral spinothalamic tract which terminates in the thalamus. Third-order neurons project to somatic cortical areas.

Fibres carrying cervical impulses are located most ventrally and medially. Thoracic, lumbar and sacral fibres are located progressively dorsally and laterally in the tract.

The *ventral spinothalamic* tract carries tactile sensation of crude touch and pressure. Its cell bodies are in the dorsal root ganglia and their axons penetrate the dorsal horns, dividing into long ascending and short descending fibres. Secondary fibres cross to the opposite side to form the ventral spinothalamic tract.

The *posterior columns* carry fibres dealing with touch requiring a high degree of localisation, vibration and position. They also carry pressure sensation. The fibres enter the dorsal column and ascend in the same side and synapse in the dorsal column nuclei (gracile and cuneate). The second-order neurons cross immediately and pass to the thalamus via the medial leminisci. Third-order neurons go to the postcentral gyrus of the cerebral cortex.

Fibres from the sacral root ganglia lie most dorsally and medially, while fibres from the cervical dorsal root ganglia lie ventrally and laterally in the posterior columns. Crossing over to the opposite side takes place in the medulla, or higher.

There are a number of *collateral* fibres. Many of these spread from dorsal column fibres to the grey matter in the initial segment where the dorsal root enters. As well, collateral fibres pass from the dorsal column nuclei to the anterior cerebellum. A few fibres pass to brainstem nuclei, and others pass to additional nuclei in the thalamus.

These collateral fibres subserve the functions of localised segmental reflexes in the cord, cerebellar reflexes that help co-ordinate motor movements, and thalamic responses which are partially responsible for the conscious perception of sensation.

The *dorsal* and *ventral spinocerebellar* tracts are concerned with proprioceptive impulses. Their cell bodies are located within the dorsal ganglia, and axons go to the dorsal horn grey matter (Clarke's columns). Here they bifurcate and pass cephalad and caudad. Secondary neurons in the column send axons to the ipsilateral spinocerebellar tract, and the fibres ascend uncrossed to the medulla and cerebellum.

## Descending Tracts

In the *corticospinal* tracts (Fig. 1) most of the motor fibres cross at the junction of the medulla and spinal cord. The fibres serving the upper extremities are deep to those serving the lower extremities. The fibres concerned with extremity movements are in the lateral corticospinal tract and those serving neck and trunk movements are in the ventral corticospinal tract. The corticospinal fibres enter the ipsilateral ventral horn grey matter and synapse with anterior horn cells. Over half the fibres terminate in the cervical cord and the remaining fibres serve the thoracic and lumbar areas.

The *vestibulospinal* tracts extend from the vestibular area of the brain in two major motor tracts descending in the spinal cord. The medial tract is limited to the cervical cord and supplies the neck and upper extremity muscles, thus

6

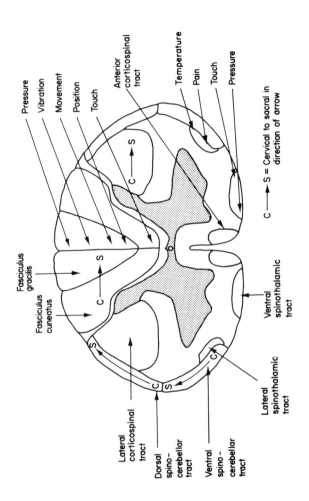

Pressure
Vibration
Movement
Position
Touch
Anterior
corticospinal
tract

Temperature
Pain
Touch
Pressure

C ——→ S = Cervical to sacral in
direction of arrow

Fasciculus
gracilis

Fasciculus
cuneatus

Ventral
spinothalamic
tract

Lateral
corticospinal
tract

Dorsal
spino-
cerebellar
tract

Ventral
spino-
cerebellar
tract

Lateral
spinothalamic
tract

Fig. 1 Principal fibre tracts of the spinal cord

helping to maintain equilibrium. The ventrolateral vestibulospinal tract descends the full length of the cord and also aids in maintaining equilibrium.

The *reticulospinal* tract systems include fibres which serve autonomic functions and are connected with the sympathetic ganglia. It also has fibres carrying important efferent respiratory impulses.

There are other spinal cord tracts whose function and anatomy are less well appreciated.

## Spinal Segments

There are 30 segments in the spinal cord, made up of 8 cervical, 12 thoracic, 5 lumbar and 5 sacral segments. In the adult, the spinal cord ends opposite the first lumbar vertebra. Hence there is a progressive discrepancy between spinal cord segments and vertebral body levels.

In the cervical area there is little difference between spinal cord segments and vertebral body levels, and the spinal roots extend from the cord almost laterally out to the intervertebral foramina. Roots C1–C7 inclusive leave above the appropriate vertebral body. Root C8 and the remainder of the spinal roots exit below the appropriate vertebral body. Although the nerve roots pass through the intervertebral foramina adjacent to their equivalent number vertebrae, the distance the roots must travel in the canal before exiting increases from the thoracic to the sacral level.

The 12 segments of the thoracic spinal cord are contained in the upper 9 thoracic vertebrae. The 5 lumbar segments are contained within T10 and T11 and the 5 sacral segments are within the canal of T12 and L1 vertebrae. The elements of the cauda equina are within the vertebral canal of the lumbar spine. The roots are so arranged that those arising at higher levels are lateral to those arising from lower levels.

Most muscles are predominantly supplied by one spinal segment, although two or three segments may contribute to its innervation. However, such muscles as pectoralis major, latissimus dorsi, serratus anterior and gluteus maximus, are true multisegmental muscles.

For ease of clinical evaluation, the following chart correlates skeletal muscles and their major spinal segmental supply:

| | |
|---|---|
| C1–3 | Neck muscles |
| C4 | Diaphragm, trapezius |
| C5 | Deltoid, biceps |
| C6 | Extensor carpi radialis |
| C7 | Triceps, extensor digitorum |
| C8 | Flexor digitorum |
| T1 | Hand intrinsics |
| T2–T12 | Intercostals |
| T7–L1 | Abdominals |
| L2 | Ileopsoas, adductors |
| L3 | Quadriceps |
| L4 | Medial hamstrings, tibialis anterior |
| L5 | Lateral hamstrings, tibialis posterior, peroneals |
| S1 | Extensor digitorum, extensor hallucis, gastrocnemius and soleus |
| S2 | Flexor digitorum, flexor hallucis |
| S2/3/4 | Bladder, lower bowel |

Tendon reflexes are each the reflex arc of one spinal segment supplying the muscle of the reflex.

| | |
|---|---|
| C5 | Biceps |
| C6 | Supinator |
| C7 | Triceps |
| L3 | Quadriceps |
| S1 | Gastrocnemius and soleus |
| S2/3/4 | Anal and bulbocavernosus reflex |

The nerves of sensation are also divided segmentally (dermatomes). There is considerable overlap of areas (Figs. 2 and 3). The following chart correlates the dermatome area and its major segmental supply.

| | |
|---|---|
| C2/3 | Neck |
| C4 | Upper shoulder and anterior upper chest |
| C5 | Lateral aspect of shoulder |

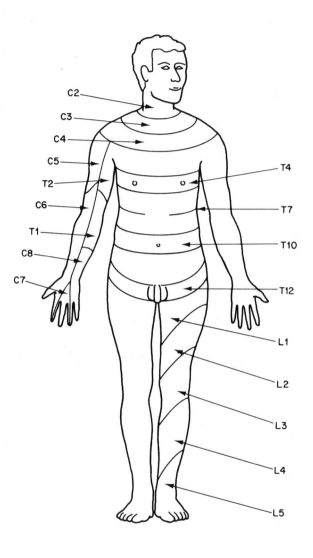

FIG. 2 Dermatomes—anterior aspect of body

10

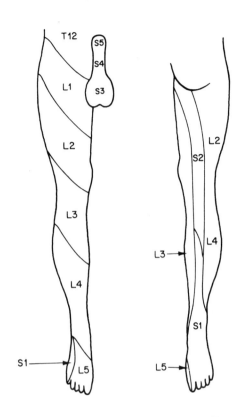

FIG. 3 Dermatomes—anterior and posterior aspect of leg and genital area

| | |
|---|---|
| C6 | Radial forearm, thumb and index finger |
| C7 | Middle finger, median strip of palm and back of hand |
| C8 | Ring and little finger, ulnar forearm |
| T1–2 | Proximal medial arm and axilla |
| T4 | Nipple line |
| T7 | Lower costal margin |
| T10 | Umbilicus |
| T12 | Groin |

11

| L1–2 | Proximal anterior thigh |
| L3 | Anterior knee |
| L4 | Anterior lower leg |
| L5 | Great toe, medial dorsum of foot |
| S1 | Lateral border foot, sole and along Achilles tendon |
| S2 | Proximal posterior thigh (narrow central band) |
| S3/4/5 | Genitals and saddle area |

Note that the dermatomes on the anterior chest go from C4 (supraclavicular nerves) to T3, C5–T2 being represented on the arm. In basing neurological assessment on trunk sensation only, it is possible to make a mistake between a paraplegic (below T3) and a quadriplegic (above T3).

SECTION 3

# SPINAL COLUMN INJURIES

It is not always possible to correlate bony column injuries with spinal cord injuries. Usually in severe disruption of the vertebral column severe neurological damage results, but not always. On the other hand, minor column disruptions usually do not cause neurological deficit, but sometimes total neurological dysfunction accompanies them.

Trauma may damage the spinal cord in the absence of bony damage by interruption of its vascular supply such as in a hyperextension injury, or by a traction effect.

The x-rays taken after a vertebral column injury show the vertebral alignment at that time. They do not indicate the amount of disruption that may have occurred at the moment of injury. They may not indicate the degree of ligamentous damage.

In children, traumatic paraplegia is rarely associated with the usual type of skeletal disruption that accompanies paraplegia in adults. In the child the skeleton is so malleable that hyperextension or hyperflexion stresses will cause a disruption of the spinal cord due to longitudinal traction or other stresses before there is any evidence of skeletal injury.

Spinal column injuries are either stable or unstable. In the former case, intact long ligaments are present and in the unstable injuries they are disrupted. In order to demonstrate the integrity of these ligaments, flexion and extension views are necessary, a risky procedure in the acute spinal patient. As such, it is wise initially to treat all injuries as unstable.

## Classification of Injuries

### Cervical Spine

*Flexion-rotation dislocation or fracture dislocation*   This is the most common injury to the cervical spine (Fig. 4), and C5–C6 is the most common site. Usually one, or both, of the posterior facets are subluxated or dislocated and may be locked in this position. There is extensive posterior ligamentous damage and these injuries are usually unstable. The spinal cord may be compressed and distracted, sustaining both direct damage and vascular damage from involvement of the anastomotic segmental vessels, or segmental feeders.

*Compression fracture*   Again C5–C6 is the usual level for this fracture (Fig. 5). The vertebral body is usually decreased in height and may be comminuted with the posterior aspect of the body encroaching upon the spinal canal. Because the posterior bony elements and long ligaments are intact, these injuries are stable. When combined with a rotation force in flexion, the 'tear drop' fracture may occur with separation of a small anterior fragment. Only about half of these injuries cause complete neurological deficit below the level of the lesion, the remainder being incomplete with the most damage to the anterior aspect of the cord.

13

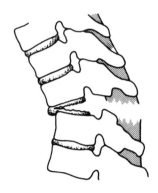 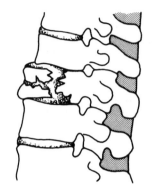

FIG. 4 Flexion-rotation dislocation or fracture dislocation of the
cervical spine

FIG. 5 Compression fracture of
the cervical spine

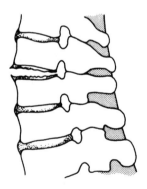

FIG. 6 Hyperextension injury of the cervical spine

14

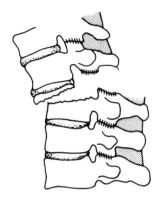

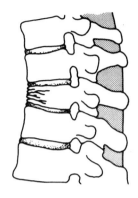

Fig. 7 Flexion-rotation dislocation or fracture dislocation of the
thoraco-lumbar spine

Fig. 8 Compression fracture of
the thoraco-lumbar spine

*Hyperextension injuries*  These injuries are most common
in the older spine with degenerative changes (Fig. 6). They
form about 30% of cervical injuries. It is most common at
C4–C5 level. Bony damage is usually not demonstrated and
the major skeletal damage is to the anterior longitudinal
ligament secondary to the hyperextension. They are stable
injuries. Most of these injuries result in incomplete cord
damage resulting from compression of the cord between the
degenerative vertebral body and disc anteriorly, and the
hypertrophic protruding ligamentum flavum posteriorly.
Summation of these forces results in central spinal cord
damage.

*Thoraco-lumbar Spine*

*Flexion-rotation dislocation or fracture dislocation*  Most of
the vertebral injuries at this level are of this type (Fig. 7).
The injury is most common at T12–L1, and results in a
forward dislocation of the upper vertebral body on the lower.
Usually there is a disruption of the posterior longitudinal
ligament, and of the posterior bony elements as well. The
inferior vertebral body usually sustains an anterior superior
wedge fracture, and some compression. These are unstable

15

injuries. Most result in complete neurological disruption either to the spinal cord, the conus, or the cauda equina.

*Compression fractures*    These injuries are common and the vertebral body is decreased in height (Fig. 8). Longitudinal ligaments are usually intact. These are stable injuries. Neurological damage is uncommon.

*Hyperextension injuries*    This is an unusual injury. It usually includes a rupture of the anterior longitudinal ligament, rupture of the intervertebral disc and an oblique fracture through the involved vertebral bodies anteriorly. These are unstable injuries. Complete spinal cord disruption is the rule.

### Open Injuries

Open injuries of the spinal column may be a result of gunshot wounds where cord damage has occurred from blast injury, vascular damage, cord penetration by the missile or by bony fragments. They are usually stable injuries with little ligamentous damage. Neurological impairment is complete in about half the cases. Stab wounds are also stable spinal injuries, incurring damage from direct penetration and vascular damage. They are usually incomplete lesions.

## Treatment of Vertebral Column Injuries

The damage sustained by the spinal cord occurs at the moment of injury. Treatment should be directed towards protection of the spinal cord from further injury at the fracture site; at the same time, an optimal environment for neurological recovery should be provided. As such then, treatment consists of reducing the bony malalignment quickly, and immobilising the injury until bony and ligamentous healing takes place.

### Conservative Management

*Cervical spine*    Traction, usually by skull tongs, is the usual form of management. This may achieve both reduction and immobilisation of the fracture or dislocation.

In dislocations where there are locked facets, manipulation under anaesthesia may be performed and the reduced position maintained with cervical traction. The fracture is then held in a suitable position of neutral, flexion or extension until healing has taken place, usually 6–8 weeks. During this time the patient is nursed on his back or on either side, being turned two-hourly. The position of traction is checked with each turn. In some centres, an electric turning bed (Keane Roto-Rest, Ireland) is used instead of two-hourly turns by a turning team.

Following traction, the patients usually wear cervical collars. High cervical fractures may require the four-poster type of collar for adequate immobilisation after traction. Collars are worn for one to two months and then flexion and extension x-rays are taken to prove stability at the fracture site. The usual type of collar does little more than remind the patient of his recent injury although perhaps they do prevent extremes of motion.

Following immobilisation by tongs, and before the patient is up and around in a collar, the neck extensor muscles are strengthened by isometric exercises.

With stable injuries of the cervical spine such as most hyperextension injuries, a cervical collar is felt to be sufficient treatment. This treatment allows the patient to be up and around. Before this, stability of the injury should be proven by flexion and extension x-rays, as some of these injuries are unstable.

*Thoraco-lumbar spine* Most injuries at this level can be managed conservatively by postural reduction in bed. Perfect anatomical reduction is not necessary to achieve a good functional result. A 6–8 week period of treatment by postural reduction is usually required for conservative treatment. Two-hourly turns are necessary during this time to prevent pressure sores. The corrective posture must be maintained during positioning on the side as well as back. This is achieved by the appropriate placement of bolsters and pillows by a turning team. After this, p.a. and lateral films usually show the bone deposited at the fracture site, and the injury is considered solid.

Before mobilisation, extension exercises are used to strengthen the back muscles. Usually movement which would tend to reproduce the injury is avoided for the first month or two of mobilisation. Then flexion and extension stress x-rays demonstrate the stability of the fracture site. At this stage the patient can go on to full programme. Back bracing is usually not necessary.

*Flexion-rotation fracture dislocations* of the thoraco-lumbar spine are unstable injuries that can usually be reduced and held by postural reduction methods. Occasionally locked facets prevent perfect reduction. In a complete neurological lesion this is of little significance.

*Compression fractures* of the thoraco-lumbar spine are stable injuries that are adequately managed by postural reduction. Because of the wedging and aseptic necrosis at the fracture site, some loss of the normal spine curve is expected.

*Hyperextension injuries* of the thoraco-lumbar spine are unstable injuries that are best managed by nursing the patient flat.

## Surgical Management

Much has been written on the indications for surgical intervention in spinal injuries. Those in favour of a surgical approach argue that until a cord is decompressed by laminectomy and the injury site seen, one cannot rule out the possibility of missing some situation that was amenable to surgery.

Some centres cool the injured area of the cord for several hours with a saline solution following laminectomy. The aim is to reduce the cord damage secondary to reactive oedema, and decrease the metabolic demands of the injured cord. The present thinking is that this is a good plan if it can be carried out immediately after the trauma.

Other efforts directed at the local area of cord damage include methods of decreasing the high levels of norepinephrine found there. Drugs such as alpha-methyl-tyrosine are effective, but too toxic for human use.

There are some situations where surgical intervention may be warranted. Any patient who has sustained spinal cord damage from an open injury such as a gunshot or a stab wound usually should have the site of damage explored to remove foreign particles, bone spicules, etc. In the patient who has a partial lesion and in whom there is neurological deterioration, exploration may be warranted to try and determine the reason for the deterioration.

Another indication for surgery is gross or late instability at the fracture site, particularly in the presence of an incomplete neurological lesion. In these cases internal fixation or grafting may be considered.

Some surgeons consider inability to achieve perfect anatomical reduction of the fracture or dislocation an indication for surgery. This incurs the risk of further neurological damage and recent comparative series show that conservative management is safer, and that the results, including neurological recovery, are marginally better.

Following surgical reduction, the patient is usually nursed on a Stryker turning frame with the usual two-hourly turns. As the fracture is reduced, positioning with bolsters and pillows is no longer necessary. Sometimes fusion is performed as a combined procedure.

Some surgeons favour early elective anterior interbody fusion, especially in cervical injuries, to achieve early stability and allow the patients to be mobilised more quickly.

Where possible, several weeks should elapse before surgery to allow traumatic oedema of the cord to settle. This gives greater assurance that the surgical intervention will not cause further neurological loss.

Myelography may be of value in pre-operative assessment. Although it indicates the level of the block in the canal, it does not allow one to distinguish between cord oedema or haemorrhage, and such mechanical things as extruded disc fragments, etc.

# SPINAL CORD INJURIES

Neural injury occurs in approximately 20% of patients who sustain injuries of the spinal column. There are varying types of spinal cord injuries, but nearly all are severe. Destruction of a small portion of the cord produces profound motor and sensory changes below the level of the lesion.

## Complete Lesions

All neurological function is lost below the level of the lesion. Paraplegia (loss of lower limb function) results from damage to the thoracic, lumbar and, to a lesser extent, sacral cord segments. Quadriplegia (tetraplegia) (loss of function in all four limbs) results from damage to cervical segments. In both conditions there is impairment of autonomic function, including bladder and bowel.

### Motor Deficit

*U.M.N.* (*upper motor neuron*)   Injuries to the spinal cord usually result in U.M.N. paralysis, characterised by loss of voluntary function, increase in muscle tone and hyperreflexia. The reflex arcs are intact but no longer connected to and influenced by central control. This loss of suprasegmental control results in a release pattern of function called *spasticity* and is found in lesions above the L1 vertebral level.

*L.M.N.* (*lower motor neuron*)   Below L1 where the cord ends as the conus medullaris, is the cauda equina. Injuries at this level and distally result in lower motor neuron paralysis characterised by loss of voluntary function, decrease in resting muscle tone, wasting and loss of reflexes. These root lesions of the cauda equina interrupt the reflex arc, and flaccidity results.

If the conus medullaris (T11–L1) is damaged, the central

20

connections of the reflex arcs for the lumbar and sacral roots may be interrupted, and this may also result in a L.M.N. lesion.

*Mixed*   A combination of an upper and lower motor neuron lesion may result from a thoraco-lumbar injury involving the conus medullaris and cauda equina. In a partial lesion at this level the intact portion of the conus and nerve roots below the lesion explain the U.M.N. part of the picture, e.g. spastic bladder and bowel (S2–S4 intact). Damage to other nerve roots will result in a L.M.N. flaccid paralysis, e.g. involving lumbar roots and resulting in flaccid paraplegia. The reverse picture can also occur.

Sometimes in spinal cord injuries of the U.M.N. type there is damage to nerve roots or root exit zones at the level of the lesion. This results in a L.M.N. paralysis of those muscles supplied by that spinal segment, and the rest of the paralysis will be of the U.M.N. type, below the level of the injury.

*Inappropriate flaccid lesions*   Occasionally an injury which usually results in an U.M.N. paralysis will result in a flaccid paralysis. This is seen most frequently in the upper thoracic lesions. The explanation for this is thought to be spinal cord infarction below the level of the lesion secondary to interruption of its vascular supply. This results in necrosis of the spinal reflex centres below the level of the injury, and a flaccid paralysis. The mid-thoracic level of the cord is the area where the blood supply of the cord is supplemented by a major segmental feeder.

*Sensory Deficit*
In complete lesions the afferent long tracts carrying the various sensory modalities are interrupted at the level of the lesion. This abolishes sensory appreciation of pain, temperature, touch, tactile discrimination and position, below the level of the lesion. Visceral sensation is also lost.

Often sensation may decrease over a few spinal segments before being lost altogether. In these cases one finds that

21

below the last normal segments there is a level of diminished sensation to pinprick (hypoalgesia) and touch (hypo-aesthesia). Distal to this there is analgesia and anaesthesia. Other patterns of sensory change below the level of the lesion are possible, in incomplete neurological lesions.

Sometimes, just at, or below the lesion, there is a level of abnormally increased sensation (hyperaesthesia and hyper-algesia). If severe enough, this is called hyperpathia.

It is possible to have differences in sensation for light touch and pain. If the spinothalamic tracts are damaged and the posterior columns are intact, as in an anterior spinal cord syndrome, there will be no pain sensation (analgesia). However light touch (normaesthesia) and proprioception will be normal, or only slightly impaired.

Some patients experience phantom limb sensations in the early period of their injury, but these usually do not persist. They may reappear, however, if amputation of a paralysed limb is performed.

### Autonomic Deficit

*Vasomotor control*  Problems with hypotension often arise in the cervical or high thoracic cord lesion—those lesions above the sympathetic outflow (T5). Because of the inter-ruption of the sympathetic splanchnic control, the upright position results in hypotension secondary to impaired venous return, and consequent syncopy. In time, adaptive mechanisms, possibly at the spinal cord level, balance this physiological problem.

The control of the vasomotor system is labile during the first few days following a cervical spinal cord injury. There is a risk of sudden cardiac arrest following routine turning of a patient at this time.

*Temperature control*  The spinal patient does not have the usual thermo-regulatory mechanisms working below the level of his lesion. This becomes especially important to the quadriplegic. His autonomic mechanisms for vasoconstriction to conserve heat, and vasodilation to lower body heat, are inoperative. He is unable to shiver and consequently is unable to increase body temperature. He cannot sweat below the level of the lesion in response to hyperthermia. Consequently the quadriplegic will tend to assume the temperature of his environment—poikilothermia.

*Bladder and bowel*   See Sections 7 and 8.

## Incomplete Lesions

In incomplete lesions there is partial preservation of neurological function. Any combination of motor, sensory and autonomic function may be spared, but these incomplete lesions usually fit into a number of recognisable syndromes.

*Acute anterior cervical spinal cord syndrome*   In this lesion the damage is mainly concentrated in the anterior aspect of the cord. The mechanism of injury may be a forward dislocation or subluxation, or compression by posterior protrusion of a vertebral body or disc. There is usually complete motor paralysis below the level of the lesion (corticospinal tracts) and loss of pain, temperature and touch (spinothalamic tracts) with preservation of light touch, proprioception and position (posterior columns—wholly or in part).

*Acute central cervical spinal cord syndrome*   In this lesion the cord damage is centrally located. The mechanism of injury is usually hyperextension of the cervical spine with compression of the spinal cord between degenerated intervertebral discs anteriorly, and a thickened ligamentum flavum posteriorly. This is most common in older men and usually there is no bony damage. There is greater damage to the more centrally lying cervical tracts supplying the arms, than the more peripherally lying lumbar and sacral segments which supply the legs and bladder. Also, the anterior horn cells supplying the cervical segments lie centrally in the grey matter and the arm paralysis may be of the L.M.N. type.

*Brown–Sequard syndrome*   In this lesion the damage is located on one side of the spinal cord, such as a hemisection

23

from a stab wound.

As a result, on the same side there may be an increased or decreased cutaneous sensation of pain, temperature and touch at the level of the lesion. Below the level of the lesion on the same side there is a complete motor paralysis (corticospinal tract). On the opposite side, below the level of the lesion, there is nearly complete loss of pain, temperature and touch, as the spinothalamic tracts cross soon after entering the cord. The posterior columns will be interrupted ipsilaterally, but as some fibres cross, this is not a great deficit. Functionally the limb with the best power has the poorest sensation, and vice versa.

*Sacral sparing*   In spinal cord injuries, the last area to be spared is the peripheral rim of tissue which is supplied via radicular arteries. This area carries sensation from the lower sacral segments. Consequently, one might have saddle area sensation in the presence of otherwise complete paralysis and loss of sensation below the lesion.

*Cauda equina lesions*   Because of the wide neural canal and the mobility of the nerve roots, cauda equina lesions are often incomplete. The mechanism of injury is usually direct trauma from fracture dislocations. The neurological sparing is unpredictable. Nerve roots may be involved either unilaterally or bilaterally. Sensory or motor loss may occur, although the common pattern is loss of both functions in a root injury. If not physically divided, nerve roots do have a potential for regrowth and recovery.

*Root escape*   A spinal injury may recover a segment or two proximally if the damage to this segment involves the nerve root and is such that the root is not divided. The recovery will be from a L.M.N. lesion at this level. These injuries are often caused by root damage at the exit foramina at the level of the spinal fracture.

*Spinal concussion*   A temporary and spontaneous reversible interruption of physiologic function of the spinal cord or cauda equina is occasionally seen in a patient who has had

24

a simple compression fracture, or perhaps no radiological evidence of injury. It is generally assumed that there is no mechanical pressure on such a cord, nor gross anatomic change within it. Another assumption is that the interruption of function is the result of a short duration pressure wave. Slow recovery indicates some reactive cord oedema.

In these patients, neurological signs regress within hours of the injury and recovery is complete in several days. Hyperreflexia in the absence of spasticity is usually seen in this syndrome.

## SECTION 5

# AETIOLOGY OF NON-TRAUMATIC SPINAL PARALYSIS

*Developmental*
Spina bifida with meningocoele, meningomyelcoele; scoliosis; spondylolisthesis; chordoma; Friedreich's ataxia and other familial paralysis; and spinal cord agenesis.

*Acquired*
> *infective:* bacterial abcess; tubercular spine; and viral (poliomyelitis, herpes, Landry's ascending paralysis and transverse myelitis).
> *degenerative:* intervertebral disc herniation; and spondylosis.
> *neoplastic:* benign (meningioma and neurofibroma); and malignant (glioma, myeloma and metastatic).
> *vascular:* A.V. malformations; angioma; dissecting aneurysm; spontaneous anterior artery thrombosis; embolism; and haemophilia and cord haemorrhage.
> *metabolic:* porphyria; and subacute combined degeneration of the cord.
> *idiopathic:* multiple sclerosis; syringomyelia; and neuromyelitis optica.

*iatrogenic :* radiation; surgical intervention; spinal injection; and vaccination.
*psychological :* conversion reaction.

# MANAGEMENT OF THE ACUTE SPINAL CORD PATIENT

## Emergency Treatment

The first aid management of patients with injuries to the spinal column and spinal cord requires the utmost caution in turning and lifting the patient so as to reduce the risk of further neurological damage.

Before moving the patient, sufficient help should be available to provide horizontal stability and longitudinal traction. Spinal flexion must be avoided. Rotation at the fracture site is also a danger when inexperienced hands are moving the patient.

It is important to try and establish the level of the spinal cord injury. The chest, abdomen and limbs must be evaluated for 'silent' lesions below the level of paralysis, such as associated chest injuries, or hidden blood loss.

Undetected sharp objects in pockets may lead to pressure sores during transportation to hospital. They must be looked for and removed.

As soon as other acute medical problems are in hand, a nasogastric tube should be passed to avoid the problems associated with vomiting due to paralytic ileus.

It must be remembered that the spinal patient is poikilothermic and will tend to assume the temperature of the environment. This is of special importance in quadriplegia. Body temperature must be preserved in cold weather, and the patient must not be overheated in warm weather.

26

Even without blood loss, the quadriplegic patient especially may present with significant hypotension. It is common to observe that the patient has bradycardia rather than tachycardia. This patient is not suffering from hypovolaemic shock, but from spinal shock due to paralytic vasodilation below the level of the lesion. Errors are frequently made in trying to correct a case of mistaken surgical shock in the spinal patient and causing problems of over-hydration. Provided the blood pressure remains above renal filtration pressure (80 mm Hg) there is no problem. The condition is usually self-limiting.

Drugs such as morphine must be used with caution in a quadriplegic who may have borderline respiratory function.

## Spinal Shock

Spinal shock refers to that state of diminished excitability of the isolated spinal cord which exists immediately and in the early stages following transection of the cord. It is also referred to as the state of 'altered reflex activity'.

This transient depression in the segments distal to the lesion is due to sudden withdrawal of a predominantly facilitating or excitatory influence from supra-spinal centres. This results in a disruption of transmission between higher centres and the synapses in the cord, and renders the process of conduction impossible.

The duration of spinal shock varies. Minimal reflex activity may appear within a period of 3–4 days but it may be delayed for up to 6–8 weeks; the average duration is 3–4 weeks. The reflex depression is more severe and lasts longer in the more proximal segments of the isolated cord than in the distal segments.

In some spinal cord patients with complete transection, sacral reflexes may be present immediately after transection. These reflexes show a delayed response and commonly disappear in a day or two. It is thought that these reflexes persist until the electrical charge remaining in the isolated cord is finally dissipated. The plantar responses are usually

27

initially absent, but may be upgoing or occasionally normal at this time. They are not a reliable sign of the presence or severity of spinal cord injury.

It has been observed that priapism occurs most frequently in complete cervical lesions, but its presence is no longer felt to be definite proof of a complete lesion.

Once the period of spinal shock has passed, afferent impulses arising from the periphery begin to elicit their excitatory influence on the isolated cord. The cord, now unrestrained by supra-spinal inhibitory influences, reacts with hyperreflexia and spasticity of the muscles. There may be motor overreaction to sensory stimuli as well as considerable radiation up and down the isolated spinal cord. Thus a sensory stimulus of the sole (S1) may cause motor withdrawal at the foot, hip flexion (L2) and even a contralateral extensor reflex.

In lesions of the cauda equina (below L1–L2) there is a L.M.N. paralysis and there will be a failure of reflex return after spinal shock. In addition, in vertical lesions of the spinal cord due to infarction or gross longitudinal traction, there will be a permanent flaccid paralysis on the basis of interruption of the cord reflex arc by the vertical spinal cord damage.

On admission, the bulbo-cavernosus and anal reflex may give a clue as to whether a thoraco-lumbar lesion will result in an U.M.N. or L.M.N. paralysis. Sacral reflexes are frequently present in an U.M.N. lesion when all other reflexes are absent. They are never present in a L.M.N. lesion.

In the spinal cord patient, if neurological recovery is to occur, signs of recovery usually appear fairly early. Patients who experience immediate total neurological loss below the lesion will probably remain complete unless they show some return of function within 24 hours. It is best to wait several weeks before giving up all hope of recovery in these cases. Incomplete lesions may recover more slowly over a longer period of time. In L.M.N. lesions, it is best to wait 3–6 months before giving up hope of recovery in complete cases as these root lesions have the capacity to regenerate if not transected, and subsequent recovery will take time. The clinical picture plus the bony damage may give a clue as to the degree of neurological damage to be expected.

## Gastrointestinal Complications

*Paralytic Ileus*

Paralytic ileus is a state of atony of the small bowel in which there is absence of normal peristaltic movement. There is a resultant accumulation of fluid and gas in the bowel.

The cause of paralytic ileus in acute spinal cord paralysis is unknown. It may be due to the sudden paralysis or subsequent metabolic changes.

This condition usually occurs after spinal cord injuries and lasts about a week, but may last for several weeks. In incomplete cord injuries it may be quite transient. The problem occurs in both U.M.N. and L.M.N. lesions.

The onset of paralytic ileus may vary. It is usually present immediately after onset of dorsi-lumbar lesions, but its onset may be delayed for up to 24 hours in a mid-thoracic lesion. In cervical lesions it may be delayed for as long as 48 hours. The reason for this variation is unknown.

The severity and period of an ileus is usually greater in patients with cervical lesions, and is more severe in complete as opposed to incomplete spinal cord lesions.

Unrecognised ileus is probably the commonest cause of sudden death in the quadriplegic patient in the first 48 hours after injury, through inhalation of vomitus. These patients are unable to cough adequately and sudden death by respiratory arrest may occur. Progressive distension of the abdomen may also cause respiratory distress in these patients by interference with diaphragmatic excursion.

A less urgent danger is the unrecognised accumulation of large volumes of fluid and electrolytes in the gut which may lead to relative dehydration, as this sequestered fluid is unavailable to the circulation. Nasogastric aspiration is imperative to reduce gut distension and reduce the risk of vomiting. Intravenous fluids are necessary for replacement, and also to feed the patient while the gut is in this non-functional state.

The end of the ileus is judged by a decrease in the amount of gastric aspiration, the presence of bowel sounds, and flatus or a bowel action.

### Acute Gastric Dilatation

The atony of the small bowel in paralytic ileus is accompanied by atony of the stomach. Uncommonly massive gastric distension occurs, sometimes caused by giving oral fluids in the presence of a paralytic ileus. This is likely to cause vomiting which may be persistent. It also causes considerable pressure on the diaphragm. Acute gastric dilatation may develop insidiously in the absence of paralytic ileus, or in the presence of an ileus. Increasing gastric aspiration or acute distension of the abdomen may be a clue to its presence. It may present as acute shortness of breath or a hypoxic respiratory arrest. X-ray will show a large dilation of the stomach shadow. It is treated by nasogastric suction and intravenous replacement fluids.

### Acute Peptic Ulceration

In 3–5% of acute spinal cord injuries, acute peptic ulceration occurs, commonly presenting as an acute gastro-intestinal haemorrhage. It usually presents suddenly 7–10 days after injury. Acute peptic ulceration is more likely to occur with severe spinal cord injuries and in spinal patients who have had acute surgery, or multiple injuries. This acute ulceration of the stomach or duodenum is thought to be due to an endogenous release of steroids after injury.

Less commonly, the ulceration may present as a perforation. This is difficult to diagnose in the spinal patient. Unexplained shoulder tip pain (intact phrenic nerve with referred pain) may be a clinical clue. An x-ray may reveal gas under the diaphragm.

Conservative treatment of the haemorrhage is indicated where possible. Blood transfusions, gastric suction and intravenous replacement of fluids is usually adequate treatment. If haemorrhage continues, an emergency surgical procedure, such as gastrectomy may be necessary.

Small amounts of blood are often present in the routine gastric aspiration of the paralytic ileus. It is not certain whether this is from irritation by the tube, or from superficial gastric ulceration. Treatment is oral antacids in frequent small doses.

*Bowel Obstruction*
The commonest cause of bowel obstruction after a spinal cord injury is from adhesions secondary to abdominal surgery for some other injury.

Occasionally a low grade sub-acute bowel obstruction is seen in the first few months after injury in the absence of prior abdominal surgery. This is probably an adynamic or functional obstruction rather than a mechanical one. It may be due to a degree of faecal impaction in a sluggish gut. It occurs most often in high quadriplegics at a variable time after injury, and may occur intermittently for a few months without any provocation. This problem presents with vomiting, abdominal distension, and increased bowel sounds. X-ray shows distension and fluid levels.

Conservative treatment should be pursued vigorously with suction, intravenous therapy, and even oil retention enemas. A surgical approach should be avoided in these cases, as they settle within 24–48 hours.

*Acute Abdomen*
The acute abdomen, either secondary to trauma in the acute patient, or as a result of perforation, or secondary to intra-abdominal infection, is difficult to diagnose in the spinal cord patient.

In the acute spinal injury, an abdominal injury with hidden blood loss may be suspected from a tachycardia and a greater degree of shock than would be expected from spinal shock alone. Plain x-rays may show free fluid or gas in the abdominal cavity. Paracentesis may confirm this. Dye contrast studies may be of help in the diagnosis of a ruptured viscus such as spleen, kidney or bladder. Pain is usually absent. Referred shoulder tip pain may be of some help when present. Abdominal guarding will be absent in spinal shock.

Abdominal pathology such as appendicitis or acute pyelonephritis is difficult to diagnose in the spinal cord patient. The symptoms will be ill-defined and poorly localised. Spasticity of the abdominal musculature makes abdominal examination difficult. Occasionally the patient might complain of an unusual feeling in the abdominal area, or tightness of the abdomen. Increased spasticity, especially initiated by examination of the trouble area, may provide a clue. Clinical signs such as temperature, pulse, respirations and blood pressure must be monitored. Rectal or bimanual examination may be of help. Routine blood work and urinalysis must always be done. It is necessary to be on the alert, for hidden pathology and routine workups will often provide the diagnosis. Very rarely would an exploratory laparotomy be necessary.

## Respiratory Management in the Acute Quadriplegic

In a cervical spinal cord lesion the injury results in paralysis of the intercostal muscles. Diaphragmatic innervation is usually above the lesion and therefore spared (C4). In a normal man, the intercostals account for over 60% of effective ventilation. It takes time before the quadriplegic develops his compensatory diaphragmatic breathing technique, and possible reflex intercostal function. During this adjustment period, the patient must be monitored for signs of hypoventilation. In cases with lesions above C4, diaphragmatic action is interfered with or abolished, and the patient will require immediate artificial ventilation.

In an unconscious spinal cord patient, intercostal paralysis may be diagnosed in a cervical cord lesion by observation of the paradoxical respiratory motion.

## Hypoventilation

Alveolar ventilation may be further impaired in a spinal patient through concurrent chest injuries or because of pre-existing lung disease.

Immediate passage of a nasogastric tube reduces the risk of vomiting and thus of aspiration pneumonia and pulmonary collapse. The tube does double duty by also decompressing a distended paralytic gut which would further compromise diaphragmatic function. In the absence of this precaution, hypoventilation may not be noted until the patient has a hypercarbic respiratory arrest.

Pulmonary oedema, due to overhydration, is avoided by strict fluid balancing. In the first days after their injury, patients tend to retain salt and water, and, if this is not realised, the patient may be overhydrated by intravenous fluids.

The cough reflex is significantly impaired due to paralysis of the intercostal and abdominal muscles. This may lead to sputum retention, infection and pulmonary collapse which will further aggravate hypoventilation. Vigorous chest physiotherapy, postural drainage and assisted coughing is effective therapy. Antibiotics are used where indicated.

Sudden respiratory arrest may occur unexpectedly following a variety of respiratory tract stimuli such as intubation, tracheostomy suction or acute bronchial obstruction by a mucous plug. It is thought this is due to reflex vasovagal inhibition, as it can be prevented by prior atropine administration.

The use of a ventilation meter will readily permit an estimate of tidal volume and vital capacity. Experience shows that, in the absence of complications, a tidal volume of 200 cc or a vital capacity of 800 cc may be adequate to maintain the quadriplegic under basal conditions.

With respect to blood gas analysis, one remembers that the slope of the oxygen dissociation curve is such that a reduction of arterial $O_2$ saturation below 90% does not occur until the alveolar oxygen tension is below 60 mm Hg—that is, until ventilation is reduced almost by half. An $O_2$ tension of 60 mm Hg is compatible with maximal physical capacity in an uncomplicated, stabilised quadriplegic. The $CO_2$ tension is a better index of ventilatory function, and serial values are helpful in following the patient. In a quadriplegic, a $pCO_2$ of under 45–50 mm Hg is usually acceptable. Plasma bicarbonate concentrations reflect adequacy of gaseous exchange, and the respiratory component of compensation in acid-base balance.

*Tracheostomy*

There are a few patients who, as a result of diaphragmatic paralysis or severe chest injury, require assisted respiration as a life-saving emergency.

In the majority of quadriplegic patients respiratory function is adequate under basal conditions. However, with consolidation, collapse or pulmonary oedema, tracheostomy or intubation may become necessary.

Some patients with pre-existing lung disease such as severe emphysema and chronic bronchitis have poor respiratory reserve even before their cord injury. With the further problems of intercostal paralysis following injury, they become candidates for tracheostomy.

Once a tracheostomy has been performed, adequate humidification of inspired air prevents a dry mucosa, tracheobronchitis and tenacious sputum. Endotracheal and endobronchial suction combats sputum retention. The suction must be carefully performed to avoid damage to the respiratory mucosa and thus provide a portal of entry for infection.

Bronchoscopy may have to be used to remove a plug of sputum causing pulmonary collapse. If so, during the procedure, precautions must be taken to avoid disruption of the spinal fracture site.

## Metabolic Management

The patient with acute traumatic quadriplegia may have a number of disturbances which stress the homeostatic mechanisms for fluid and electrolytes.

Respiratory acidosis may be a complication of hypo-ventilation and $CO_2$ retention.

Nasogastric suction may result in an alkalosis associated with a loss of gastric HCl. Acidosis may complicate loss of small intestinal secretions from suction, or loss internally by sequestration in the gut.

In the post-traumatic period, probably because of enhanced mineralocorticoid activity, the patient is likely to have a positive sodium balance. Infusion of sodium chloride solutions may result in pulmonary oedema, and the chloride overloading stresses the buffer system. If such is the case, it may be necessary to promote a diuresis using 20% mannitol, as fluid overload presents a grave danger in the acute quadriplegic with already compromised respiratory function.

There is increased loss of potassium in the urine, also due to mineralocorticoid action. Such potassium deficits may be large and their restoration may require intensive therapy—up to 300mEq/24 hours may be necessary in the intravenous fluids. Failure to provide adequate potassium during the acute period will delay the restoration of smooth muscle function and hence the paralytic ileus will be prolonged. Cardiac irregularities may also develop.

The fluid and electrolyte regime, using a physiological electrolyte replacement fluid, and dextrose and water preparation, is directed to cover gastrointestinal loss, replace urinary and insensible loss, and impose a minimal electrolyte load on the kidney. Urinary output should be 2–3 litres per day. Within the first 10 days a post-traumatic diuresis must be watched for and appropriate fluid adjustments made.

The average patient has a basal caloric requirement of 1500–2000 kcal/day. With inadequate caloric intake, the body glycogen stores are rapidly depleted in the first day, and a negative nitrogen balance and starvation ketosis results. This, plus a metabolic acidosis, may require a bicarbonate infusion to correct the buffer system.

Calories may be provided in several forms in I.V. therapy. Fructose is less likely to cause thrombophlebitis in concentrations over 5% than glucose, and is more easily metabolised. Ethyl alcohol is a good caloric source, is a mild sedative and combats thrombophlebitis by its local vasodilator effect. Insulin may be used to facilitate carbohydrate metabolism and promote potassium and amino acid uptake by the cells. Simple sugars like fructose and sorbitol do not cause as much stimulation of endogenous insulin production as a regular diet.

Synthetic amino acids may be given to spare body proteins. The patient must have a good caloric intake before these amino acids will be utilised efficiently.

By using these replacement fluids and additives, it is possible to maintain fluid electrolytes and acid–base balance, avoid or repair starvation ketosis, provide the high-energy substrate necessary for tissue repair, and convert the negative nitrogen balance to a positive one.

## Venous Drainage Complications

*Deep Vein Thrombosis*
The incidence of clinical thrombosis is similar to that of non-paralysed post-surgical patients. Diagnosis by venography reveals a much higher incidence.

There are three main factors which encourage thrombosis in the spinal patient. Firstly, there is considerable stasis in the venous system due to loss of muscle pump action. Secondly, local trauma to the paralysed legs results in damage to leg veins; this is abetted by the continuous contact of the calves and thighs with the bed. Prolonged immobilisation is the third factor.

As well, there is some lowering of arterial blood pressure, particularly in the higher lesions, but this is compensated for to some extent by the decreased arterial peripheral resistance due to vasomotor paralysis.

The patient does not complain of pain. There will be swelling of the involved limb, local rubor and temperature rise, and a slight systemic temperature rise. A thrombosis of the inferior vena cava will result in bilateral signs. In an

36

U.M.N. lesion, spasticity may be noted to increase, especially in the afflicted limb. Diagnostic procedures are usually not necessary, but when required, venography is a useful test to delineate the level of the venous thrombosis. Doppler flow techniques and isotope studies can also be used.

The tendency to develop venous thrombosis may be reduced by a twice-daily full range of passive movements of the lower limbs to promote venous drainage. Established thrombosis may be treated with elevation, bed rest and crêpe bandaging. The latter procedure may run the risk of circumferential pressure sores if improperly done. Anticoagulants are not without risk in a patient who has an indwelling catheter, and their use is directed by the severity of the clinical condition. Some centres use them prophylactically in all new patients.

## Pulmonary Embolus

This is the serious complication of deep vein thrombosis and is one of the causes of sudden death in the early weeks. Fortunately, as a serious clinical entity, it is uncommon. Small pulmonary emboli may pass unnoticed. The fatal ones are usually large, and often bilateral.

In the spinal patient, acute onset of respiratory distress may be the presenting picture, with tachycardia, pyrexia and rapid respirations. In high lesions pain will be absent.

Chest x-ray, looking for wedge-shaped infarcts, may be helpful in large infarcts, or a small pleural effusion may be seen in lesser ones. E.C.G. evidence of right heart strain may be present. Friction rubs may be auscultated. Where available, radioisotope pulmonary scans are useful when used serially to diagnose and follow the infarct.

Usually, immediate treatment with anticoagulants is sufficient to control this problem.

## Gravitational Oedema

Due to loss of assistive muscle pumping action for venous drainage, gravitational oedema is a problem in the spinal patient. The oedema is more common and severe in flaccid L.M.N. lesions. U.M.N. lesions have some muscle pumping by virtue of their spasticity. The problem is more common in older patients with incompetent venous valves.

In most patients, the oedema is a problem when they first begin to mobilise from bed when their fracture is stable. After they have been up in their chairs for a few weeks, a local homeostasis prevails. Local muscle tone improves as does local vasomotor tone, and the oedema is not as much nuisance. Elevation and/or elastic stockings are usually sufficient treatment.

The differential diagnosis must include cardiac failure, deep vein thrombosis, heterotopic bone formation and pathological fracture. With elevation, the gravitational oedema disappears overnight. With the other causes it does not.

## SECTION 7

# THE NEUROGENIC BLADDER

Prior to World War II, most spinal patients died within a few years of their injury, and usually from a renal cause. Since that time, due to the improved care of the urinary tract, spinal patients live almost normal life spans, and less than half die from renal pathology.

### Normal Bladder

*Anatomy* Bladder musculature consists of a syncitium of smooth muscle which cannot be divided into layers. The fibres are so arranged that when the detrusor contracts, the vesical neck is simultaneously pulled open by muscle fibres which insert into the prostatic urethra in the male, and the entire urethra in the female. As the bladder neck is thus opened, the ureters are pulled inferiorly, thereby aiding in the prevention of vesicoureteric reflux.

The internal urethral sphincter has not been demonstrated anatomically. Continence is maintained passively by the intrinsic tone of the smooth muscle and fibroelastic tissue of the female urethra, and the prostatic urethra in the male.

In the male there is a definite external urethral sphincter composed of the striated muscles of the urogenital diaphragm. In the female these structures are not present, but there is striated muscle at least on the anterior surface of the female urethra. Whether this functions as an external sphincter is in dispute.

*Neuroanatomy*    The reflex control of micturition resides in the sacral 2–4 spinal segments. Parasympathetic fibres leave in the pelvic nerve (nervus erigentes) and proceed to the bladder where they synapse. Somatic nerve fibres also leave the S2–S4 segments in the pudendal nerve and usually supply the perineal muscles including the external urethral sphincter. The somatic nerve supply plays no direct role in continence. Its role seems to be voluntary interruption of the urinary stream when voiding. Sympathetic nerve fibres arise from T11–L2 cord segments and pass to the sympathetic chain, and then on in the hypogastric nerves to the bladder, prostate, seminal vesicles and proximal urethra. The sympathetic nervous system plays no clear role in the control of micturition, although sensory fibres are known to run from the bladder with the sympathetic fibres.

*Physiology*    When the bladder is filled (approximately 400 ml), sensory afferents in the sympathetic, parasympathetic and somatic divisions are stimulated and transfer impulses to the micturitional reflex centre of the cord. The desire to void and sensation of fullness reaches the brain through the posterior columns. Cerebral control provides an inhibitory influence to reflex micturition.

After the inhibitory effects of cortical control are released, motor impulses descend via the corticospinal tracts then travel via the parasympathetic fibres to the bladder.

Increased detrusor tone results, shortening of the trigone with closure of the ureteric orifices, and opening of the internal urethral orifice. This is accompanied by voluntary relaxation of the perineum and contraction of the abdominal wall and diaphragm. The bladder empties. If desired, the stream can be voluntarily interrupted by contraction of the perineal muscles.

## Neurogenic Bladder

The neurogenic bladder is one whose function has been modified by some interference with its nerve supply. After a spinal cord injury, the effect on the bladder depends on the time interval after injury, the level of cord injury and the degree of cord damage.

During the period of *spinal shock*, the areflexic, flaccid paralysis below the level of the lesion includes the bladder function. The patient will develop acute retention with overflow incontinence. A catheter is required.

In *U.M.N.* lesions, reflex activity returns as the phase of spinal shock passes. In a lesion above the conus, the spinal micturitional reflex arc is intact, and an automatic type of bladder results. The bladder will empty involuntarily as it fills with urine. The capacity may be less than normal, but there is good voiding pressure at capacity. There is no sensation of bladder fullness.

In *L.M.N.* lesions, the spinal micturitional reflex is interrupted and an autonomous bladder results. Bladder function is governed by a myogenic stretch reflex inherent in the detrusor fibres themselves. This type of dysfunction is characterised by a linear increase in intravesical pressure with filling until capacity is reached. Urine then may flow past the sphincter by overflow incontinence.

In mixed *UMN–LMN* lesions, such as with a conus-cauda equina injury, it is possible to have a flaccid LMN detrusor, and yet a spastic sphincter. The reverse may also occur.

Other patterns of mixed neurogenic bladder may occur

with incomplete cord lesions where there is partial voluntary control overriding reflex function. Precipitate urination results. This is common in central cord syndromes and Brown–Sequard syndromes.

## Bladder Training

*Investigation*
After the period of spinal shock, and before bladder training is intensified, a bladder profile is obtained through several tests.

The bulbocavernosus reflex and anal reflex are tests of perineal somatic nervous supply. The former is elicited by rapidly squeezing the glans, or tapping the clitoris, with the examining finger in the anus. The normal response is contraction of the anal sphincter. The anal reflex consists of the contraction of the anus following a scratch of the perianal skin.

The autonomic supply of the detrusor can be checked by the ice water test. 50 ml of sterile water is instilled into the bladder through a straight catheter. If the reflex is intact, the water and catheter will be expelled immediately.

All these reflexes return early in the UMN lesion. After spinal shock, their absence indicates a LMN lesion.

The cystometrogram is a helpful guide to the type of bladder present, and its capacity. Using a simple water manometer one is able to plot volume capacity against intravesical pressure. If room temperature solution and a slow drip infusion are used, an accurate account of bladder capacity and voiding contractions can be plotted. In a normal bladder there is a gradual intravesical pressure rise, first desire to void is felt at 200 ml and a voiding contraction (40 mm $H_2O$) takes place at about 400 ml. In the UMN bladder, intravesical pressure will rise more sharply and there will be intermittent contractions while it fills. Finally a precipitous voiding contraction of large magnitude will empty the bladder. In LMN lesions, the intravesical pressure rises slowly, there are no contractions, and voiding

41

is usually by overflow. Mixed bladders will show a combination of these pictures.

An I.V.P. is done routinely to serve as a base line of renal function and to delineate the collecting systems. Blood urea and creatinine are also used to follow renal function.

A voiding cystogram, or retrograde introduction of dye into the bladder, is used to outline the urethra (urethrogram) and bladder (cystogram) looking for diverticulae, etc., to indicate bladder capacity and to demonstrate vesicoureteric reflux if present.

Cystoscopic examination is used to inspect the bladder mucosa, the outlet area, and for stone identification and removal.

*Early Bladder Management*

The general aims are to achieve a catheter-free state wherein the bladder consistently empties completely, the urine is sterile, and the patient remains continent.

During spinal shock there are no reflex contractions of the detrusor. In this period, the detrusor should be exercised by allowing the bladder to fill to capacity inter-mittently. This can be done by two-hourly catheter clip-offs twice a day, for the patient with an indwelling catheter. It can also be achieved by twice-daily distension with an antiseptic bladder washout solution for the person with an indwelling catheter. Tidal irrigation may be used to maintain volume capacity.

Alternatively, intermittent catheterisation may be per-formed. Initially the catheter is passed 6 times per 24 hours, and fluid intake is strictly monitored to 150–200 ml per hour. Fewer catheterisations are needed as the patient begins to pass urine with efforts at voiding. Excellent results regarding the number of patients attaining catheter-free states with sterile urine can be expected. One to 3 months after injury for patients on an intermittent regime is a reasonable time estimate for return of detrusor activity, compared to 3–6 months for those treated with indwelling catheters.

## Upper Motor Neuron Bladder

In the UMN bladder on catheter drainage, detrusor training can be intensified with two-hourly clip-offs through the day, and straight drainage through the night. During this time the patient learns the relationship between fluid intake and urinary output. He learns to substitute a time clock for the lost feeling of the desire to void.

With the catheter removed, the UMN bladder must be stimulated to initiate the reflex detrusor contraction and to empty efficiently. The reflex contractions occurring spontaneously from the filling of the bladder usually do not empty the bladder completely. The spinal patient finds a 'trigger point' to augment the voiding contraction. The patient thus learns to empty his bladder at least every 4 hours for the rest of his life. If he forgets and lets the bladder partly empty itself reflexly, the bladder will become over-distended and more difficult to empty completely. The residual urine will predispose to infection. Reflux with ascending infection and pyelonephritis may occur.

Drugs can be used to supplement detrusor training. Those that facilitate parasympathetic function may be used to improve reflex contractions. Carbachol is the best of this group, but Urecholine, although weaker in action, causes fewer side effects of parasympathetic over-activity. To decrease the detrusor spasticity which may be excessive Probanthine may be used. It is also of help in controlling autonomic hyperreflexia.

## Lower Motor Neuron Bladder

In the LMN bladder on catheter drainage, detrusor training is usually begun with two-hourly clip-offs to maintain bladder capacity and detrusor tone.

Although the LMN bladder is denervated, the detrusor has some inherent contractile ability. As long as the bladder does not become chronically distended for long periods of time, this contractile force can be utilised in bladder emptying. Volume control is important when trying to utilise this contractile force. There is an optimal length/tension ratio for detrusor fibres. Beyond a certain length, the fibres do not work efficiently. As such, if the LMN bladder distends to too great a volume, it will be difficult to empty effectively.

With the catheter removed, this type of bladder can only be emptied by external pressure. This is done by increasing intra-abdominal pressure by straining if the abdominal musculature is intact, or by the Crede manoeuvre where direct pressure is applied to the bladder by manual suprapubic pressure.

Drugs like Carbachol and Probanthine have little use in LMN bladder training as the reflex arc is not intact and the bladder is denervated.

### Other Neurogenic Bladders

Incomplete lesions often demonstrate loss of cortical inhibition so that many uninhibited bladder contractions take place, most of which occur at low pressure, but which finally develop true voiding pressure with resultant precipitate micturition. Probanthine is helpful in damping these contractions and allowing the patient greater warning before micturition.

### Residual Urine

It is necessary to train the forces of expulsion to overcome the resistance of the bladder neck outlet. Once voiding is possible, then a balance between expelling forces and outlet resistance must be achieved so the bladder is able to empty, or very nearly so.

In bladder training, residual urine determinations are a useful test of bladder function. Much of the time spent in training is used in trying to reduce the level of residual urine. Efficient emptying techniques must be developed. Drugs like Carbachol may be helpful in augmenting detrusor reflex emptying. High residuals predispose to reflux, back pressure on the kidneys, as well as persistent urinary infection and stone formation.

*Collecting Devices*

Once off the catheter, males usually use some type of incontinence device for collecting urine, such as a condom or urosheath apparatus draining into a leg bag, as the majority of patients are incontinent of urine even though they have a balanced bladder.

Occasionally problems arise with a short shaft of penis or redundant foreskin which allows the sheath to slip off even when firmly taped on. The latter problem can be dealt with by circumcision.

There are also firmer rubber urinals into which the penis fits, and which can be reused after cleansing. Stoke Mandeville and Bard–McGuire are two of these. Abrasive areas on the penis from the firm rubber, pressure areas from the suspending straps, and difficulties with erections are some of the problems with this type of drainage device.

No satisfactory collecting device has been developed for female patients. It could be this fact which motivates females to achieve a higher 'off catheter and continent' success rate than males. Another explanation for this may be in the different pelvic floor musculature of the female. The patient must be able to go at least 2 hours between emptying times to make the off-catheter regime socially practical. Because of these difficulties a greater proportion of women require permanent indwelling catheters than men.

*Outlet Obstruction*

Outlet resistance in patients with UMN lesions is common and complex. The internal sphincter does not contribute to outlet obstruction. Its function seems to be the prevention of ejaculation of semen into the male bladder. Obstruction is usually caused by a spastic external sphincter. Proof of this may be obtained by a pudendal nerve block which will temporarily paralyse the external sphincter by blocking its nerve supply. This block may provide continuing relief by allowing urine to pass, which further stretches the sphincter. If the result is only temporary, repeat blocks or nerve section may be tried. The disadvantage of the latter is that it

45

permanently interrupts the sacral reflex arc and may remove the ability to have penile erections in the male.

The commonest surgical procedure for relief of external sphincter spasm is external sphincterotomy, performed transurethrally. It appears to be most effective when combined with a T.U.R. prostate.

In a LMN bladder, the absence of reflex function leaves the prostate as the only potential source of obstruction. Prostatic hypertrophy is unlikely in the young patient. Inefficient voiding technique is the common explanation for high residual urines in this group, rather than outlet obstruction.

### Balanced Bladder

A balanced bladder is one where the residual urine is consistently low. The absolute value of the residual urine volume is not as important as its percentage of the voided volume, within certain limits. The usual aim is to achieve a repeatable residual urine of about 10% of the voided volume, although 20% in LMN bladders is acceptable. The actual residual should not be over 50 ml.

Bladder balance usually takes 1–3 weeks after the removal of the catheter for a trial of voiding. Some patients never achieve it. One of the factors preventing a bladder from becoming balanced is a poor bowel habit with impaction. For this reason trials of voiding are usually not commenced until the bowels are fully trained. This usually delays bladder training in paraplegics, as the bowels cannot be properly trained until the patient can get on and off the toilet himself.

Cystitis and calculi are other foci of irritation which may increase the bladder and sphincter spasticity in an UMN bladder, and make balancing difficult. Also, pressure sores, foci of infection and anxiety can significantly contribute to bladder spasms.

Finally, if bladder balance is prevented by excessive spasticity radiating from the legs which has proved refractory to conservative treatment, it may be necessary to treat this spasticity first by some destructive procedure such as intrathecal alcohol blocks or rhizotomy, thus converting an upper motor neuron bladder to a lower motor neuron bladder.

## Complications of Catheter Drainage

*Catheters*
There are three types of urinary catheters in general use. The commonly used catheter is the soft rubber Foley type with an inflatable retention balloon, usually size 14–16F. These require weekly changes. The Silastic catheter is of similar design, coated with a silicone substance. The suggested advantage of these is that they are inert, therefore causing less infection and calcium aggregation. They may be left in place for up to 5 or 6 weeks.

The Gibbon catheter may be used in the male. It has the advantage that it is both of small diameter (size 6–12) and made of fairly inert plastic so that it is less irritating than the larger Foley. The Gibbon has no retention balloon, but is strapped to the penis via its plastic flange. It is useful in males for the first few weeks after the onset of paralysis until it becomes blocked by debris or is bypassed as a result of bladder spasms. It is not necessary to change it until it becomes blocked or the patient develops urethritis.

In intermittent catheterisation a small bore red rubber catheter is used. As sterile technique is used and the catheter is not left in place, infections should not accompany this method of drainage.

Catheters must be strapped to the abdominal wall when *in situ*. This will prevent periurethral abcesses and pressure necrosis at the angular portion of the male urethra at the penoscrotal junction, and secondary formation of diverticulae and fistulae at this level. Such complications may require suprapubic diversion of urine and direct surgical repair, and the results are often successful.

Suprapubic catheters should be mentioned to be con- demned as a routine method of bladder management. Their use is confined to drainage during surgical procedures, as mentioned.

*Infection of Urine*

With the use of an indwelling catheter, the urine will eventually become infected. With good technique it is possible to delay and minimise infection. The technique of catheterisation is especially important and it should be regarded as a sterile surgical procedure. It is also important to irrigate the urethra with an antiseptic 1:5000 chlorhexidine solution before passing the catheter, as the urethra normally harbours organisms that will cause infection if introduced into the bladder. Another source of infection of urine is from upward spread in the catheter; therefore sterile containers are used for urine collection.

A problem with the Foley catheter is that the balloon of the catheter lifts the drainage hole in the catheter tip away from the most dependent part of the bladder. This allows a stagnant pool of urine to collect at the base of the bladder which may result in infection and stone formation. A high fluid intake (3 litres per day) helps minimise this risk. Manual bladder washouts may be necessary.

Occasionally the low-grade localised bladder infection may become blood borne or reflux up the ureter and cause acute pyelonephritis. This diagnosis is largely clinical, the patient being febrile, having rigors, nausea, etc. The presence of pyuria or bacteruria is not sufficient for this diagnosis in the catheterised bladder.

Epididymitis is a common complication in males on catheter, probably secondary to retrograde infection via the vas deferens, and the stasis caused by the *in-situ* catheter. Recurrent epididymo-orchitis in a patient on long-term catheter drainage may necessitate ligation of the vas deferens.

Antibiotics are not used routinely or prophylactically in a patient on catheter drainage. These patients usually show some urinary growth of bacteria. The routine use of antibiotics in the presence of a catheter will not eradicate the urinary bacteria, only change the organisms and increase

48

their resistance to antibiotics. The urinary bladder somehow establishes a local relationship with these bacteria. In the absence of a high residual urine or reflux, their growth is partially controlled by and confined to the bladder, and no systemic effects result.

Whether on the basis of chronic infection or not it is unknown, but the incidence of bladder carcinoma in long-term spinal patients is much higher than in the normal population.

A patient on catheter drainage who shows systemic signs of ascending urinary tract infection should be promptly treated with appropriate antibiotics until asymptomatic.

Once off the catheter, every attempt should be made, using antibiotics, to produce a bacteria-free urine.

*Bladder Calculi*

These may be a problem in catheterised patients with complete cord transections. They induce irritability of the bladder and a general increase in spasticity. They are usually radio opaque, having a high calcium content, and can be seen on an abdominal plain film.

The spinal patient has a hypercalcuria secondary to mobilisation of skeletal calcium associated with paralysis and immobilisation. This predisposes to stone formation. Efforts to reduce calculus formation include a high fluid intake and restriction of milk and other dairy products. Routine urinary acidification with Mandelamine, and ascorbic acid or ammonium chloride helps prevent stone formation. This lowers the urinary pH to around 5 and discourages aggregation of calcium salts which form best in an alkaline medium. However, when the 'mycin' antibiotics have to be used, these acidifying drugs must be stopped and the urine alkalinised to enhance the activity of the antibiotics.

Stones form around a nidus, and infection provides such a nidus. Chronic urinary infection has a high association with calcium phosphate stones. Control of urinary infection is important, and this is best achieved in the catheter-free state. 'Egg shell' calculi tend to form around the retention

49

balloon, another good reason for getting rid of the catheter.

Not only stasis of urine, but stasis of the patient is also a potent factor in stone formation, so measures to encourage patient activity are important in minimising hypercalcuria secondary to immobilisation osteoporosis.

Most bladder calculi can be treated by transurethral crushing and removal. In the treatment of renal calculi, conservation should be practised. Ureteric stones pose a problem in that they are often silent and present with secondary infection. Their management is no different in spinal cord patients than in non-paralysed patients.

*Other Complications*
Unskilled catheter changes may be the cause of serious problems other than infection. Forceful introduction of the catheter may lead to formation of false passages and the risk of perforation.

Inflation of the balloon while the catheter tip is still in the membranous prostatic urethra, may cause significant haemorrhage or urethral rupture.

The bladder on long-term catheter drainage without clip-offs will contract and become increasingly spastic with trabecular hypertrophy and diverticulae. These present problems with voiding past the catheter because of the small capacity and increased spasticity. Once present, the small capacity bladder may be resistant to increases in its capacity and may need to be managed surgically by a bladder by-pass procedure.

*Autonomic Hyperreflexia*
Blockage of the catheter in a patient with a lesion above T6 (sympathetic outflow) may lead to autonomic hyper-reflexia. It may also be precipitated by visceral distension from a full bowel, stimulation of the skin secondary to an irritative pressure sore, and vesicoureteric reflux. Labour in the high-quadriplegic pregnant female may also be complicated by it. Blocked catheter with bladder distension is the commonest cause.

The usual clinical signs are bradycardia, sweating, rhinorrhoea, pounding headaches, and severe paroxysmal hypertension. The syndrome presents quickly and can rapidly precipitate epileptic fits, cerebrovascular accidents and death if not relieved.

The mechanism is as follows: impulses produced by any of the previously mentioned stimuli are transmitted through the pelvic and pre-sacral nerves to the spinal cord. From there, via the lateral spinothalamic tracts and posterior columns, the impulses ascend to the level of the cord lesion. Here a sympathetic reflex is activated and results in massive reflex sympathetic nerve over-activity below the level of the lesion. There is arteriolar spasm in the skin and viscera, increasing peripheral resistance and resulting in hypertension. This stimulates pressure receptors in the carotid sinus and aorta. The centres respond via the vasomotor centre within the brainstem with vagal stimulation and consequent bradycardia. Impulses from the vasomotor centre which would cause splanchnic pooling and allow a decrease in blood pressure are blocked at the level of the cord lesion. Consequently hypertension and bradycardia persist until the cause of the autonomic crisis is removed.

If the site of irritation is the bladder, after drainage is re-established the installation of local anaesthetic will block the afferent arc of the reflex. Systemic Probanthine may also help in damping afferent stimuli from irritated visci.

It may be necessary systemically to reverse the hypertension by administration of ganglionic blocking agents such as diazoxide (hyperstat).

*Vesicoureteric Reflux*
Vesicoureteric reflux of any significance is a serious complication of the neurogenic bladder. This most often occurs after the acute management period, often months or years after. It is more often present in patients with UMN bladders than in those with LMN bladders. The presence of reflux may be a contra-indication to spontaneous voiding.

51

Reflux cannot be considered an insignificant complication because the mortality from uraemia is three times higher in spinal patients with reflux than in others. Recurrent pyelonephritis in combination with raised back pressure is the mode of renal tissue destruction.

Long-term catheter drainage may be indicated in situations such as vesicoureteric reflux, hydroureter and hydronephrosis. With careful management and good technique, patients can be managed on long-term catheter drainage without progressive renal decompensation. Figures are now available showing twenty-year periods of successful catheter drainage in spinal patients. This is under optimal circumstances, but with poor catheter management, chronic infection, stone formation and repeated illness is the common situation.

Upper renal tract dilatation is a secondary complication of reflux. If chronic infection is also present, a surgical approach for urinary diversion may be used rather than long-term catheter drainage. This involves implanting the ureters into an isolated loop of bowel (ileum or colon) which has an opening, or stoma, on the abdominal wall. Continence is provided by an adhesive appliance. The loop is not designed to store urine, but rather it is a conduit by-passing the bladder and so draining the upper tracts freely.

This procedure is a major undertaking and there is the possibility of urinary and bowel leakage, bowel obstruction and urinary obstruction at the anastomotic sites. Subsequently most careful attention to stoma and appliance is essential for satisfactory function. The bladder which has been defunctioned may cause problems with local sepsis and require intermittent antibiotic washouts, or even removal at a later date.

Another surgical technique involves bringing the dilated ureters to the abdominal wall to make a satisfactory stoma (cutaneous ureterostomy). This may result in ischaemia of the ureter, or a stenosis at the stoma may occur, defeating the purpose of this drainage procedure.

*By-passing*
Patients with indwelling catheters occasionally experience voiding around the catheter. Usually by-passing occurs in a spastic bladder which is being irritated by a noxious focus, such as infection or stones. Anything that increases somatic spasticity tends to increase bladder spasm and results in by-passing. A small-capacity spastic bladder will also result in by-passing.

Treatment of this condition consists of diagnosing and treating the reason for the by-passing—usually an irritative focus of some kind. It is not sufficient to replace the urinary catheter with one of a larger size. This only results in urethritis, possible urethral diverticulum formation and continued by-passing.

## SECTION 8

# THE NEUROGENIC BOWEL

### Normal Bowel Function

Incontinence of faecal matter through the anus is prevented by tonic contraction of the internal anal sphincter (smooth muscle) and the external anal sphincter (striated voluntary muscle).

Ordinary defaecation results from the defaecation reflex: with faeces in the rectum, distention of the rectal wall initiates afferent signals that spread through the myenteric plexus to initiate peristaltic waves in the descending colon and sigmoid, forcing faeces towards the anus. As the peristaltic wave approaches the anus, the internal anal sphincter is inhibited by receptive relaxation, and when the external sphincter is voluntarily relaxed, defaecation occurs.

The defaecation reflex is extremely weak, and to be effective it must be fortified by another reflex involving the sacral cord segments. When the afferent fibres in the rectum are stimulated, signals are transmitted into and back from the sacral cord by parasympathetic nerve fibres (nervi eregentes from S2–S4). They greatly intensify the peristaltic waves and make the defaecation reflex effective. Also, the afferents entering the cord initiate other effects of increasing intra-abdominal pressure by straining which forces the faecal matter distally.

Control of defaecation is achieved by voluntary control of the external sphincter (pudendal nerve from S2–S4). This is a skeletal muscle which is kept tonically contracted when preventing defaecation. When this is done, the defaecation reflex diminishes and does not return for several hours.

This reflex can be initiated by abdominal straining, but reflexes produced this way are not as effective as those that arise naturally.

## Neurogenic Bowel

In a spinal cord patient with a lesion above the sacral segments the defaecation reflex is intact, but will cause automatic emptying of the lower bowel because normal control exercised through voluntary contraction of the external sphincter is lost, and sensation is impaired or lost. This somatic sphincter will be hypertonic or spastic in the UMN lesion.

In a LMN lesion, the reflex is interrupted but the autonomous bowel still has some intrinsic contractile response of the smooth muscle, probably mediated by the myenteric plexus locally. The external anal sphincter is patulous in the LMN lesion.

## Bowel Training

In the acute or early stage, some prefer the use of para-sympathetic stimulants such as Prostigmine to get the gut working. Usually this is not necessary, as the smooth muscle peristalsis will begin as soon as the ileus secondary to spinal shock disappears.

54

Whether the cord lesion is UMN or LMN makes little difference in bowel training, except that the UMN lesion with its tonic external sphincter may be a little easier to regulate.

In bowel training a fixed time pattern takes the place of the cerebrally monitored urge. The defaecation reflex is initiated by local anal stimulation using suppositories or rectal touch technique. In the UMN patient, advantage is taken of the intact reflex by initiating it at a time of convenience for bowel emptying, thus preserving continence. In a LMN lesion with no sacral reflex present, continence is assured by a regularly evacuated bowel. In this case, a faecal load and suppositories stimulate the local smooth muscle reflexes for emptying.

The usual pattern is an every-other-day evacuation. This is preceded by night-before laxatives or detergent stool softeners, and triggered by suppositories. The time chosen for evacuation should take advantage of the post-prandial gastrocolic reflex. A good diet with sufficient bulk is necessary for the production of well-formed stools. Hydrophilic substances may be used to provide soft bulk. Patients usually work out a satisfactory bowel habit by trial-and-error, finding the emptying time and the amount of laxative and suppositories that best suit them.

Once this routine has been established, it is usually reliable and the patients do not have bowel accidents. It is important to avoid anything which may upset the habit, such as change of diet, poor fluid intake, drugs such as Codeine or change of bowel emptying time pattern.

Occasionally when the pattern has become irregular, the patient will become impacted. One of the earliest signs of this is overflow faecal incontinence or increased somatic spasticity. The usual method of dealing with this problem is oral stool softeners or laxatives, and disimpaction as well as repeated enemas until the low bowel is clear. Then the patient's own bowel pattern should be started again.

A common error made by patients after discharge from hospital is deliberate constipation in an attempt to prevent bowel accidents. This will usually produce more frequent accidents through faecal impaction.

High faecal impaction in the quadriplegic may present with a picture of obstruction with distension. X-ray will show a dilated lower bowel with fluid levels, and a lot of faeces. These cases respond to conservative measures of nasogastric suction and fluid replacement, and the use of oil retention enemas. Surgery should be avoided as this condition clears in 24–48 hours.

Sometimes faecal impaction may reflexly cause bladder dysfunction. Correction of the impaction cures the bladder complaints.

Most paraplegics and some low quadriplegics will be able to transfer to the toilet for management of their bowels. With high quadriplegics, the bowel treatments may be administered in bed by an attendant, or better still, in a commode chair over the toilet pan.

## SECTION 9

# PRESSURE SORES

### Pathophysiology

The cause of these lesions is pressure. Bed sores and decubitus ulcers are simply pressure sores incurred in the recumbant position.

There is a definite pressure/time relationship in the production of pressure sores. Skin can tolerate a minute pressure indefinitely, whereas a great pressure for a short time produces disruption. Between these extremes there is a spectrum of pressure versus time which may cause a pressure sore. With usual pressures from body weight, microscopic tissue changes secondary to local ischaemia can be seen in less than 30 minutes. Experience has shown that these

56

changes are reversible if pressure does not persist for more than 2 hours.

On the microscopic level, pressure can be seen to interfere with arteriolar and capillary blood flow, and therefore tissue nutrition. Local anoxic changes result. There is a build-up of local tissue metabolites from interference with venous blood flow. Oedema develops, further embarrassing tissue nourishment. These ischaemic changes result in tissue death. Besides a direct pressure force, there is usually a shear force in the tissue interfaces which further interferes with tissue perfusion.

Clinically, various stages can be distinguished in the evolution of a pressure sore. As a result of transient circulatory disturbance, pressure causes redness of the skin without tissue destruction. This redness disappears with the removal of pressure. With prolonged pressure, there is a definite superficial circulatory and tissue damage. This may be associated with congestion and induration of the area, or blistering and loss of the superficial epidermal layers. With more pressure, the deeper skin layers are lost which leads to superficial necrosis and ulceration. After a high pressure force, or prolonged pressure, there results deep penetrating necrosis including skin, subcutaneous tissue, fascia and muscle, leading to local gangrene. This destruction may include underlying bony structures. Osteomyelitis with sequestrum formation may result.

Pressure necrosis can begin from within, usually in an area over a bony prominence. A sterile abcess forms and slowly surfaces, only then revealing the extent of tissue destruction.

Bony prominences tend to concentrate tissue pressure from body weight as the relative pressures are much greater over these small areas.

During spinal shock there is a relative tissue hypoxia secondary to loss of vasomotor control and decrease in the rate of peripheral circulation. This contributes to a lowering of tissue resistance. Other than during spinal shock, the only factor that renders the spinal patient more liable to the development of pressure sores is his deprivation of his sensory warning mechanism—not an inherently greater liability to tissue breakdown. In addition the skin of the aged, anaemic and hypoproteinaemic patient does not have a greater tendency to breakdown than an average patient. These debilitating factors may decrease his activity and therefore cause prolonged pressure resulting in pressure sores. Once present, a pressure sore will heal slowly in such a patient.

Macerated or unhygienic skin provides fertile ground for pressure sores as the skin nutrition and blood supply is already compromised. For the same reason these factors interfere with healing.

Following the development of one pressure sore, unskilled nursing efforts to avoid pressure in this area often result in pressure areas on the opposite side or over the sacrum. To heal bilateral or multiple pressure sores requires the specialised nursing techniques of a spinal unit.

With formation of a pressure sore, the serous drainage constitutes a continuous loss of protein. This can amount to as much as 50 grammes a day.

The chronic sepsis of a pressure sore may affect the haemopoietic system resulting in a normochromic, normocytic anaemia. With long-term sepsis there exists the risk of secondary amyloidosis.

## Treatment

*Prophylaxis*
Frequent cleansing of the skin with soap and water and brisk drying removes the macerated skin and skin oils, and cleanses skin pores and hair follicles. The drying stimulates local circulation. This is a good local defence against pressure sores. The use of spirits as prophylaxis is to be condemned.

Water beds, ripple mattresses and other devices have been used in an attempt to minimise the pressure which is taken by vulnerable areas of the body. They do not prevent pressure sores if the main requirement of frequent and regular changes of posture is neglected. In the wheelchair, the spinal patient must develop the ritual of relieving sitting pressure for a short time at least twice an hour.

In the prevention of pressure sores, there is no place for the use of air rings or 'doughnuts'. These are liable to produce tissue death by circular occlusion of the blood supply.

The spinal patient should inspect his body each evening with the use of a mirror to watch out for early signs of pressure sores. For the rest of his life this pressure consciousness must continue.

*Conservative Management*
The patient should be put at rest in such a manner that the ulcerated area will bear no further pressure. Excision of devitalised tissue and evacuation of an abcess should be undertaken. With adequate drainage and local toilet thus guaranteed, the way is clear for the formation of healthy granulation tissue. Antiseptic solutions such as Eusol, etc. are best used for frequent local cleansing. Frequent changes of dry dressings avoids the complication of maceration from antibiotic impregnated gauze.

Depending on the severity of the lesion, systemic antibiotics may have to be used after blood and local cultures have been taken. Local antibiotic creams are of little use. The usual chronic anaemia is best treated by transfusion. This combined with a high-protein high-carbo-hydrate diet will much improve healing powers.

For the more superficial pressure sores, antiseptic cleansing and dry gauze dressings will suffice. Many pre-parations are variously advocated, some as simple as sugar dressings, others as splendid as gold leaf. Vitamin E ointments or cortisone preparations are suggested for epithelial cell stimulation. With due respect, good hygiene and pressure relief are sufficient to ensure healing. One can put anything on a pressure sore, except the patient, and it will heal.

## Surgical Management

For those pressure sores which extend deep into muscle or bone, and involve large areas, surgical closure may offer the most expedient cure. Surgery must never be contemplated until all conservative measures have been instituted and the wound is clean, pink and lined with healthy granulation tissue. At this juncture, instead of awaiting healing by second intention, closure may be advocated.

Repair by excision and direct closure may be possible if closure can be effected without undue skin tension. The surrounding scar tissue is excised together with any dead bone. A thick layer of tissue is directly approximated thus achieving linear closure. Haemostasis is important and suction drainage is often used post-operatively.

When it is impossible to approximate wound edges, closure may be achieved by fashioning a flap of skin and subcutaneous tissue, and swinging it over the wound. This provides a durable, full thickness repair which is especially important over a bony prominence. The secondary defect is repaired by a split skin graft.

Split skin grafting is suitable for superficial sores where there is an adequate layer of subcutaneous padding over underlying bony prominences.

Pressure on the site of repair should be avoided until healing is complete. When the patient is turned, it is important to avoid movements which will cause pulling on the wound.

It is important that no stress be placed on the wound for a minimum of 3 weeks. It is desirable to wait 6 weeks before a patient sits directly on an operative scar, but this depends on the exact site and nature of the scar. The patient must understand that the site of repair will not resist further pressure injury as well as previously intact skin. It is important that there is a graduated increase in sitting time on a newly healed area.

The healing of a serious pressure sore is a tedious process. Months of careful nursing attention are required. The expense of time and money to the community is enormous.

It is a great inconvenience to the hospitalised patient who really is not 'sick'. For all these reasons there is no treatment for pressure sores that is superior to prevention.

# SEXUAL FUNCTION IN THE SPINAL CORD PATIENT

## Normal Physiology

Sexual function in the male is a complex interaction of spinal cord reflex function, supra-spinal influences as well as hormonal and psychological factors.

The spinal reflex arc concerned in sexual function has peripheral afferents, spinal cord centres and peripheral efferents.

The peripheral afferent stimuli are light touch carried by the pudendal nerve (somatic S2–S4) and pressure carried by the pelvic splanchnic nerves (parasympathetic from S2–S4).

There are several centres in the cord serving the sexual functions of erection, seminal emission and ejaculation. There are two centres for erection, a 'reflexly activated centre' (parasympathetic S2–S4), and a 'centrally and psychologically activated centre' (sympathetic T11–L2). The seminal emission centre is sympathetic at T11–L2. The centre for ejaculation is somatic S2–S4.

There are three peripheral efferent pathways. The parasympathetic (S2–S4) centre sends fibres in the pelvic splanchnic nerve 'nervi eregentes' supplying the corpora cavernosa and prostatic gland, and giving rise to erections and formation of seminal fluid. The sympathetic (T11–L2) centre sends fibres in the hypogastric nerve supplying vas deferens, seminal vesicles and prostatic muscles giving rise to seminal emission. There are also some cholinergic fibres

61

to the corpora cavernosa which give rise to erection. The somatic centre (S2–S4) sends fibres in the pudendal nerve to the bulbospongiosus and ischiocavernosus muscles as well as the pelvic floor, giving rise to ejaculation.

There are also supranuclear pathways concerned with the spinal reflex system. Afferent spinal tracts carrying impulses of light touch and friction are transmitted in all three spinal columns. Proprioceptive impulses are transmitted in the posterior columns. These impulses all eventually reach the cortex. Central afferent fibres carrying olfactory and visual impulses reach the cerebral cortex and subsequently the sympathetic and parasympathetic nuclei of the hypothalamus. Efferent spinal tracts carry somatic efferent impulses in the pyramidal tracts extending to the anterior horn cells. Visceral efferents from the hypothalamus travel to spinal preganglionic cells in the thoraco-lumbar lateral horn and the sacral sympathetic preganglionic cells.

## Sexual Function in the Male Spinal Patient

Generally speaking sexual function in the male spinal patient will depend on the level and completeness of the lesion. In complete lesions there usually is loss of function dependent on supraspinal and cerebral centres such as psychic erection and orgasm, and, to a lesser extent, effective ejaculation and seminal emission. Lesions above the reflex centre in the conus (UMN) retain the ability of reflex erections secondary to cutaneous stimulation of the glans penis, but there will be no sensation with sexual intercourse.

In some low cord lesions above the sacral reflex centres, the patient may not only have reflex erections, but also psychogenic erections. These occasionally may be accompanied by ejaculation. Emission is often precocious, but rarely associated with orgasm. This phenomenon is felt to be mediated via an intact sympathetic nervous system.

In incomplete UMN lesions there is a variable ability to have psychic erections, ejaculation and orgasm, but the chances are greater than in complete lesions.

In LMN lesions such as a cauda equina transection, the ability to have a reflex erection is lost. Occasionally these patients may be able to have psychogenic erections if the sympathetic pathways are intact, but this is extremely variable. The psychic erections are frequently followed by precocious emissions and, if accompanied by an orgasm, it is not of normal acuity. The LMN patient will occasionally have a seminal emission or even ejaculate without erection.

If the LMN lesion is incomplete, the patient is more likely to have psychic erections than reflex erections, followed by emission accompanied by an orgasm-like sensation.

The spinal patient is often able to have adequate erections to achieve satisfactory intercourse as far as the couple is concerned, though he may not have any sensation of his genital organs himself. The psychological factors of being able to satisfy his mate play an important part in intercourse, and this is often a reasonable substitute for lack of genital sensation. The female may assume the role of aggressor and the dominant position during intercourse.

The important thing to remember is that any form of sexual practice that is satisfactory to both partners and is within the bounds of their moral and social code is correct for them. Understanding the problems and experimentation in this area should be encouraged.

In spinal cord males overall, erection is achieved in 75%, coitus in 35%, and ejaculation in 10%.

## Reproduction

The ability to sire children is much reduced in the spinal patient. This may be due to several factors: inability to have erections, inability to ejaculate or retrograde ejaculation into the bladder, or an inefficient seminal emission. Other less-understood causes include chronic infection in the prostatic urethra, repeated epididymo-orchitis resulting in obstruction or destruction of testicular tubules, and impaired spermatogenesis.

In spinal cord males overall, less than 5% sire children. The percentage of progency is poorest in complete UMN lesions, about equal for incomplete UMN and complete LMN, and highest in incomplete LMN lesions. These figures may be altered in the future by the technique of intrathecal injection of Prostigmine or rectal electrode stimulation of prostate and vas deferens. These methods produce a reflex erection and simultaneous ejaculation. The ejaculate is collected, and if adequate numbers of motile spermatozoa are observed, auto-artificial insemination may be performed.

## Sexual Function in the Female Spinal Patient

The female is much better off than the male as far as sexual function is concerned, either in the patient with an UMN or a LMN lesion. In the complete lesion, other than lacking genital sensation, sexual function is unimpaired. Satisfaction during intercourse is usually derived from being able to satisfy the male partner.

## Pregnancy

Fertility is unimpaired by the cord lesion. Pregnancy is usually normal. Uterine contractions occur quite normally in the female spinal patient and therefore labour is usually normal, with the advantage of painless contractions. The absence of secondary powers of expulsion such as abdominal contraction does not seem to impair labour.

There are a few points to note concerning the spinal patient in labour. In the absence of painful contractions, labour may advance more quickly than is realised, and a precipitous delivery may ensue.

In a patient with a high level of paralysis the possibility of autonomic hyperreflexia during labour must be watched for. This must be managed with ganglion blocking drugs, or caesarian section.

Another difficulty may be the bladder. In the later months

of pregnancy, a balanced bladder is likely to come un-balanced with the increasing size of the uterus, and catheter drainage may be required. In addition, childbirth often stretches the bladder neck and interferes with the balanced bladder. Some feel it is worth doing an elective caesarian section to preserve good bladder function. The decision for an elective caesarian section has to be worked out individually for each case.

## SECTION 11

# SPASTICITY

### Physiology of the Stretch Reflex

The stretch reflex is essential in maintaining muscle tonus and providing a background of postural tone against which voluntary movements can occur.

*Afferent Arc*
Stretching a muscle stimulates specialised receptors—its muscle spindles. These are encapsulated organs containing intrafusal fibres, which carry two distinct sensory organs. These spindles have a parallel arrangement with the extrafusal muscle fibres.

In the first type of intrafusal muscle fibre sensory organ, there is a collection of nuclei in its central region called the *nuclear bag*. It is this region which carries the primary sensory ending, an annulospiral arrangement. These conduct impulses to the spinal cord along the fastest afferent fibres (IA fibres). The nuclear bag intrafusal muscle fibre has its own motor supply through small myelinated gamma I fibres.

The second type of intrafusal muscle fibre sensory organ is the nuclear chain fibre. In its central region it con-tains a chain of nuclei and it is around this region that the primary ending is wound. It conducts impulses along the IA fibre. It also carries a second ending which transmits impulses along a group II afferent, and thence to the spinal cord. The motor innervation of the nuclear chain fibre terminates in the same region as the secondary sensory ending. These motor fibres are derived from small myelinated gamma II fibres, and they end in a thin axon trailing along the muscle fibre.

Besides the muscle spindle, which detects the length of extrafusal fibres and their rate of change, there are receptors in tendons called Golgi tendon organs. They detect tension during contraction and transmit information to the motor control system of the spinal cord and cerebellum. They cause reflexes associated with damping of muscle movements, with equilibrium and posture. Their signals are transmitted through rapidly conducting A alpha fibres.

Internuncial cells are present in the base of the dorsal horn, and are spread diffusely in the anterior horn of the spinal cord. The interconnections between internuncial cells and anterior motor neurons are responsible for many of the integrative functions of the cord. Most incoming sensory signals are first transmitted through internuncial cells. These interconnections can modify signals tremendously.

*Efferent Arc*

The large fibres from the primary receptors go directly to anterior motor neurons and cause monosynaptic reflexes. Others transmit signals to the cerebellum. The fibres from the secondary receptors terminate on the internuncial cells and elicit more delayed patterns of reflexes.

Signals from the Golgi tendon organ are felt to excite an inhibitory interneuron that in turn inhibits the anterior motor neuron.

The parallel arrangement of intrafusal muscle spindles and the main muscle mass provides activation of spindle discharge by passive stretch, and interruption of spindle discharge by active muscle contraction.

The gamma loop refers to the circuits to and from the spinal cord involving the muscle spindle with its gamma efferent fibres. The muscle spindle may be considered the sensing element of a reflex system which registers differences in length between itself and the main muscle mass, and acts to reduce the difference. The role of supraspinal controls on the gamma system can be facilitory or inhibitory.

## Spasticity

Following spinal shock in UMN lesions there is a gradual increase in tone of the paralysed muscles, and involuntary movements begin to appear. This continues until there is hypertonus, hyperreflexia and clonus. The explanation is excessive reflex activity below the level of the lesion. The reason for this is thought to be release from supraspinal inhibitory impulses from the brain.

The muscle spindle responses are particularly hyperactive, probably due to gamma motor neuron discharge. Overactivity of gamma I motor neurons leads to increased phasic stretch reflexes. Overactivity of gamma II is responsible for increase of static stretch reflex activity.

The average time for the appearance of spasticity is about 6 weeks in cervical injuries and about 10 weeks in thoracic injuries. Usually reflex excitability is at a maximum about 2 years after the spinal cord injury and gradually diminishes. The development of spasticity may erroneously be interpreted as return of function.

Almost all cervical spinal cord injuries have spasms. 75% of thoracic lesions have spasms. Less than 58% of lumbar lesions have spasms and less than 25% of conus-cauda equina lesions produce spasms. Partial lesions may have more severe spasms than complete lesions. As well in incomplete lesions, voluntary motor function can be seriously overridden by spasticity and make the voluntary function useless.

There tend to be two main patterns of spasticity—flexor and extensor. The statement that flexor spasticity occurs with complete cord lesions and extensor spasticity occurs with incomplete lesions is untrue. Either or both patterns can usually be demonstrated in complete and incomplete UMN lesions. The type of spasticity that develops in a patient is dependent upon the stimulus applied to the paralysed part. A poorly nursed patient tends to develop flexor spasticity, while a patient who is better positioned and more active, especially if walking, will tend to develop an extensor spasticity.

The danger of untreated or excessive spasticity is the development of contractures, especially with flexor spasticity of the antigravity muscles. After a time the muscles involved shorten, and there is a fibrous contracture of the muscles and the joint capsule, greatly reducing the range of motion. These contractures may make positioning and personal hygiene difficult. Alternatively, excessive extensor spasticity can eject a person out of bed or from a wheelchair, leading to injury.

Generally speaking, spasticity is a nuisance to the spinal patient. It does help in some ways by maintaining muscle bulk, improving lower limb circulation and decreasing osteoporosis. Some patients are able to trigger spasticity of an otherwise useless muscle and utilise this in trick movements. Some can use extensor spasms of the legs in standing transfers. However, when excessive, spasticity can be troublesome, and must be dealt with when it interferes with normal patient activity.

## Treatment

*Prevention*

The physiotherapist plays an important role in minimising spasticity. It is essential that the paralysed limbs are put through a full range of motion at least twice daily. This is combined with passive stretching of spastic muscles.

As an extensor pattern of spasms is of more functional benefit, efforts are made to suppress a flexor pattern and develop more of an extensor pattern. In bed, efforts are made to prevent a flexed attitude. The upright posture encourages the extensor pattern so, where practical, standing and walking are encouraged.

Irritating foci below the level of the lesion are sought and corrected as they contribute to an increase in spasticity.

Anxiety leads to a generalised increase in spasticity which is both difficult to explain and hard to treat. Patient psychotherapy with the help of anxiolytic drugs is a good approach to the problem.

### Conservative Management

*Physiotherapy*  The rationale for the technique of passive movements is to fatigue the stretch reflex of a spastic muscle as well as to maintain range of movement. Hydrotherapy may be used as an adjunct to physiotherapy. Some claim warmth relieves spasticity, others use cold. It tends to vary in individual patients.

*Drugs*  Drugs may play a part in management, but the problem cannot be overcome by drugs alone. The most useful drug to date is Valium (Diazepam) which has a direct depressing effect on polysynaptic reflexes. The exact site of action is unknown, but most agree it has a specific antispasmodic effect on striated muscle.

*Nerve blocks*  The simplest nerve block is of peripheral nerves. This is useful in spasticity confined to a particular muscle group. Phenol or alcohol may be used. Unfortunately, spasticity often then becomes a problem in an associated muscle group. Another approach is to combine a temporary block using local anaesthetic with physiotherapy.

*Motor point blocks*  By using diluted phenol solutions instilled in motor end points, the smaller, more vulnerable gamma motor fibres may be blocked, making the muscle spindles less sensitive to stretch. Because the larger fibres are not affected, voluntary motor power will not be affected. The effect is temporary, lasting from weeks to months.

*Subarachnoid blocks*  For generalised excessive spasticity of legs, a phenol or alcohol subarachnoid block may be used. This converts an UMN lesion to a LMN lesion by demyelination of the treated spinal roots. The problem is that bladder and bowel function may be impaired, and any sexual function will be lost. It cannot be used in incomplete lesions, as it will destroy any residual function. Alcohol usually has a permanent effect, phenol less so.

### Surgical Management

*Neurectomy*    This is the simplest procedure for spasticity, where the peripheral nerve is interrupted. Obturator and pudendal neurectomy are the more common procedures done. This creates a LMN lesion of supplied muscles.

*Rhizotomy*    For more generalised spasm, anterior or posterior nerve roots can be divided in the spinal canal. This has the advantage of being selective, and sparing sacral root function if desired.

*Myelotomy*    The Bischoff myelotomy may be performed for generalised lower limb spasticity. It surgically divides the connections between anterior and posterior horns, thus breaking the reflex arc. It is technically difficult.

*Chordotomy or chordectomy*    These are rarely used.

*Orthopaedic procedures*    Division or lengthening of the tendons of spastic muscles is done to decrease the amount of spasticity without abolishing it. The principle is to increase the length–tension ratio and put the muscle at a disadvantage by elongation. Adductor tenotomy, hamstring tenotomy and Achilles lengthening are common examples.

SECTION 12

# ASCENDING MYELOPATHY

Traumatic spinal cord paralysis is usually a stable condition, that is to say in its chronic state it does not progress.

Post-traumatic syringomyelia provides the exception to this rule. In less than 2% of spinal patients there is a progressive loss of higher spinal cord function. This tends to occur after a variable time lapse. In complete lesions the average time lapse is less than 5 years, while in incomplete lesions the time lapse is greater than 10 years.

The signs and symptoms reflect an asymmetrical grey matter spinal cord syndrome. It has a history presenting with pain, or occasionally numbness, and then loss of function. The process begins unilaterally involving pain and temperature fibres, reflex fibres, and occasionally anterior horn cells. If the myelopathy descends, it may present as a changing picture of inappropriate flaccidity below the level of the original lesion. This would be explained on the basis of interruption of reflex arcs. Descending lesions are much less frequent.

This condition seems to be caused by the formation and progressive expansion of a cyst or syrinx in the grey matter. How this cyst begins is not known.

On myelography, the involved cord segment may appear widened in diameter. Cord central canal dye studies may demonstrate the cavity.

Surgical procedures which drain or shunt the cysts may arrest this condition, and may even result in some regression of signs.

SECTION 13

# CHRONIC PAIN

## Aetiology

In the acute spinal patient, pain at the site of injury to the spine is present for only a few days. This pain is caused by torn ligaments and fractured bones, the most severe pain being due to local muscle spasm in this region.

In the chronic spinal patient, pain is of a different aetiology and nature. True anaesthesia, meaning lack of sensation, is practically non-existent. There are many sensations below the level of the lesion, most of which are unpleasant. They follow bizarre patterns and seem to encompass all sensory modalities. There are usually no obvious causative factors for these intrinsic feelings. The pain is diffuse and imperfectly localised. In some centres it is reported in over 90% of patients, disabling in 30%, and intolerable in less than 10%. Severe pain seems to be greatest in cauda equina lesions, but in these cases, there might be a mixture of this plus root entrapment pain.

It is suggested that the site of origin of this pain is the distal end of the proximal segment of the interrupted cord. This is postulated because spinal anaesthetics failed to alter the burning pain.

Another type of pain may occur at the level of the injury and is due to a lesion of the spinal nerve roots. This pain may be avoided by proper reduction of the bony injury, or relieved by decompression of the involved roots.

Pain may also occur secondary to instability of the fracture site, and may necessitate a spinal fusion. Unfortunately this procedure, even when orthopaedically successful, is not always successful in relieving pain.

In the anxious spinal patient, pain may be a common complaint necessitating an outpatient visit. After the anxiety-causing problems have been identified and discussed, this pain seems to diminish proportionately.

## Treatment

The *physiotherapist* has an important role in prevention of pain by minimising painful contractures and reducing spasticity by stretching.

*Reassurance* by the medical staff, with an explanation of the cause of the pain, is important in treatment of this problem.

*Drugs* should not be used for the diffuse non-localised

72

type of pain. Occasionally they may be necessary for root pain. The patient who is incapacitated by his pain will be the one who will quickly become drug dependent.

*Nerve blocks* can be used in diagnosis of root pain and as a form of conservative treatment. In general, alcohol permanently destroys neural tissue, while phenol tends to have a less permanent effect.

*Local infiltration* of local anaesthetic and corticosteroids into painful paraspinal areas may be helpful in relieving discomfort. They should be followed by physiotherapeutic mobilisation of the area.

*Surgery* has a small but definite place in the relief of chronic pain. A specific neurectomy or root section may be performed to relieve local pain. Posterior rhizotomy may be necessary for the chronic pain which may accompany a cauda equina lesion, in an effort to relieve the pain, but spare the sacral segments. For severe pain below the level of the lesion, a tractotomy may be necessary, with division of the spinothalamic tracts.

Recently a dorsal column stimulator has been successful in relieving chronic pain, presumably by interruption of ascending pain afferents.

SECTION 14

# PARA-ARTICULAR HETEROTOPIC OSSIFICATION (P.A.O.)

Laying down of bone around a joint is a fairly common complication of paralysis, probably occurring in 15–20% of all spinal patients.

The cause is unknown although local trauma such as from vigorous stretching is often suspected but not proven. The hip is the commonest joint involved, followed by knee, elbow and shoulder, in that order.

73

Calcification occurs first in between muscle layers, not in muscles as with myositis ossificans. However, elevation of C.P.K. laboratory values suggests participation of skeletal muscle. Calcification is followed by immature bone and finally mature bone formation results.

Clinically, P.A.O. may present as a localised warm swelling in the vicinity of a joint. There may be palpable induration or diminution of passive range of motion. Serial x-rays will document the evolution of bone formation.

Treatment should be conservative. Maintenance of a good range of motion in the involved joint is achieved by gentle passive movement.

Occasionally the new bone will limit function to such an extent that the bone must be removed. Experience has shown that the bone will recur if removed before it is mature. It often takes 18–24 months for bone maturation to occur.

Elevation of alkaline phosphatase indicates growing bone and is a contra-indication to surgery. Elevation of hydroxy-proline levels has been noted during development of this heterotopic bone, but normalisation of these levels does not necessarily mean that the bone has matured. Serial bone scans seem to be the best way of deciding when the bone is mature, and thus the optimal time for surgery.

## SECTION 15

# OSTEOPOROSIS AND PATHOLOGICAL FRACTURES

In a spinal patient there is marked osteoporosis of the bones in the paralysed extremities. In the quadriplegic, because of partial voluntary movement, the arms are involved to a lesser degree than the legs.

This phenomenon is a type of disuse osteoporosis, but is more marked. It begins immediately after onset of paralysis, and the loss of protein and calcium salts occurs most rapidly in the first few weeks. Thereafter homeostatic mechanisms tend to slow the process, and eventually a new equilibrium is reached. It is this loss of calcium from bone and its excretion in the urine which is mainly responsible for the development of bladder and renal calculi in spinal patients.

The osteoporosis is more marked in the flaccid LMN lesion. In the UMN lesion, spasticity maintains muscle tone and provides involuntary movements which preserves more of the bone substance.

Pathological fractures occur secondary to this osteoporosis. They occur most commonly in the leg bones, particularly the femur. A common site is the supracondylar region. The trauma resulting in fracture may be minor, a careless transfer, fall from a wheelchair, or physiotherapy being common causes.

The diagnosis may be made on the basis of local swelling, pathological mobility and crepitus. Spasticity may be increased locally. X-ray confirms the diagnosis.

Treatment should be conservative whenever possible. Pillow splints may be used effectively. Healing occurs rapidly even though the bones are osteoporotic.

If internal fixation or plasters are necessary, the dangers of pressure sores must be kept in mind and suitable precautions taken.

Skin traction is contra-indicated. Skeletal traction is not often used because of the pressure sore risk to the leg and the sacral area.

## SECTION 16

# AIMS IN REHABILITATION

The general theme of rehabilitation in the spinal cord patient is to make maximum use of the remaining function.

The general goal is the highest degree of independence permitted by the neurological lesion. A successful rehabilitation programme should bring the patient to the level where he is again able to work. Some say the successfully rehabilitated patient is one who pays income tax.

## Paraplegia

During the acute management in bed, efforts are made to maintain and improve upper limb strength, as well as strengthening any other surviving muscle groups.

Muscle strength is graded as follows:

Grade 0—no movement.

Grade 1—visible or palpable motion.

Grade 2—strength sufficient to move the adjacent joint through a complete range of motion in a gravity eliminated position.

Grade 3—strength sufficient to move the joint through a complete range of motion against gravity.

Grade 4—as Grade 3, but with the ability to overcome some resistance as well.

Grade 5—normal strength.

These tests should be done three times in a row through the full range, before the result is determined.

Once out of bed, the strengthening is carried on so that wheelchair mobility will be maximal. Competent balance in and out of the wheelchair is also stressed. Transfers to bed, car and shower or bath are practised. One tries to instil confidence in the chair to the point where it is regarded as a part of the whole patient.

Dressing and toileting are further goals in the A.D.L. programme. Car driving is usually necessary because of the great difficulty in using public transport.

T2–T12 lesions should be fully independent in the wheelchair and management of A.D.L., including bladder and bowels. The better the thoracic innervation, the better the sitting balance.

T12 and below lesions have the realistic possibility of walking with calipers and crutches. They have at least the advantage of hip hikers, the quadratus lumborum. Although higher thoracic lesions can be fitted with braces, the work required for walking is too great to make it practical. Surveys show that patients with lesions above T12 do not persist in walking after discharge. They may use the braces and crutches for standing as part of a daily home physiotherapy programme. It is not surprising that they cease walking, as their energy requirement is similar to that of a normal man running up several flights of stairs.

The more musculature present across and below the hips, the more chance the spinal patient has of becoming a successful walker. L3 and below lesions may be able to walk with just short leg braces and crutches, depending on the strength of the quadriceps.

## Quadriplegia

The same general strengthening and balancing programme is carried on with quadriplegics although the goals for independence of locomotion and A.D.L. are limited by the severity of the lesion.

In a summary form, lesions below:

C4—upper extremity function can be carried out only with the use of externally powered devices.

C5—with assistive devices the patient will be able to feed himself, perform some grooming activities, use a typewriter, push a wheelchair slowly, and help with dressing. He will be dependent in transferring, bladder and bowel care. Electric wheelchair may be necessary for longer distances.

C6—the presence of wrist extensors for a tenodesis grip makes grasp and release possible. Should be able to dress, handle wheelchair more efficiently and transfer with an overhead trapeze. The patient will probably need some assistance with bowel and urinary appliances.

C7–8—the presence of finger flexors and extensors makes hand activities possible without assistive devices. The presence of triceps makes transfers feasible. Wheelchair independence is possible.

T1—the patient has normal arm and hand function and therefore is a high paraplegic. Balance will be poor, being mainly dependent upon the latissimus dorsi.

In rehabilitation, progress is often rapid in the early stages, but levels off in 4–6 months. The standard of independence achieved depends entirely on the way a patient works and his desire to achieve.

# PSYCHOLOGICAL PROFILE OF A SPINAL PATIENT

## General

Although there is no such thing as a spinal paralytic personality, one does see a large number of young men who have common psycho-social backgrounds. They come from lower socio-economic strata, there has been a lack of discipline in their lives, they have left school at an early age, and their jobs and pleasures are both physical and dangerous.

Once the injury has happened, this person must enter an entirely new world. He must learn to take responsibility for his own complete care, he will no longer have the luxury of physically aggressive outbursts, and he will have to approach life in an organised and efficient manner.

## Immediate Reactions

*Anxiety, depression* There are usually several phases of emotional ups and downs during the period of rehabilitation. Clinically the reactions of anxiety and depression are seen as soon as the patient has recovered from the immediate effects of his injury. Sometimes these reactions are delayed or disguised. Discussions with the patient about what his condition means to him, what his expectations of treatment are, and his future plans will often precipitate a confession of anxiety and depression. These discussions do far more in the treatment of the problem than Valium or mood elevators.

*Denial* When a newly paralysed person does not seem to be depressed, usually what is happening is a denial of functional loss or of its social implications. Denial can be a useful temporary solution, but it becomes a problem if it persists as a significant mechanism.

*Grief, mourning* Another immediate reaction to spinal paralysis is that of grief and mourning behaviour. These patients need time to mourn their loss of body function. Time is, to a large extent, the healer.

*Somatic fears* The obvious changes in body function are a great source of concern to the patient. In excretory function, especially during retraining, great tensions and anxieties arise. When a bladder or bowel accident occurs, the patient feels responsible and guilt and shame are aroused. The attending staff must realise this and explain the situation to the patient, and try to put him at ease.

Sexual function, or the lack thereof, haunts the young male spinal patient. Worries of sexual performance are closely integrated with his feelings of manliness. Proper explanation of the situation and what the patient can expect in the future helps to reassure him.

## Long-Term Reactions

A prominent form of adjustment is dependency. There are two general types: overdependence and underdependence.

*Overdependency*   The overdependent patient will seek approval, demand a lot of staff attention, ask excessive questions, be fearful of trying new things, and show inability to make decisions. This represents a sense of being overwhelmed by the catastrophe without the hope of being able to get hold of things. Time will help some of these patients. Others regard the injury as their 'out' from the competitive world. They feel they no longer should be required to be self-reliant and self-supporting.

*Underdependency*   The underdependent patient will be inappropriately confident, obstinate, unable to accept appropriate offers of help, and will set unrealistic goals. Too much of reality is being denied for this patient's ambitions to be sustained over a long period of time.

*Aggression*   Other patients will have an aggressive behaviour pattern. Although it is irritating to the staff, counter-hostility should be avoided, as then personal antagonism becomes a problem. At least this type of patient is fighting his disability, albeit inappropriately. Efforts should be made to constructively redirect this aggression.

*Somatic complaints*   The chronically anxious patient will often present time and again with functional increases in his symptomatology. These are somatic manifestations of his fears. The best treatment is patience, and reassurance. The patient must be made to feel that people do care and are interested in him. As he begins to understand this, his functional complaints will subside.

The goal of rehabilitation is always directed towards promoting ego integrity and feelings of self-worth. The aim is to assist the person towards reforming a self that approves of continuing life, despite the discontinuity with his past identity. The patient must develop a new self-image based on feelings of self-worth.

# MORTALITY

Before World War II, few spinal patients survived more than two years. If they survived beyond the acute stage, they usually died of the complications of chronic urinary sepsis and pressure sores.

Now, where adequate care is available, early mortality is less than 10%. The long-term life expectancy for paraplegics is an average of 10% less than the normal population, and 15–20% less for quadriplegics. The reason for this change is medical care which prevents or adequately treats complications of spinal paralysis, rather than any dramatic advancement in specific treatment of the paralysis.

### Early Mortality

*Chest complications*   An acute death is one occurring within 2 months of the onset of paralysis. Chest complications of collapse, consolidation and pneumonia in the absence of adequate chest physiotherapy, pulmonary oedema secondary to fluid overload and inhalation of vomitus are the chief causes of death in the acute period. These deaths are largely preventable.

*Multiple injuries*   The next common cause of death is that from the combined effects of multiple injuries. The precise cause of death is unknown, but probably metabolic failure contributes. This cause of death is not attributable to the spinal injury *per se*.

*Haemorrhage*   Massive acute gastrointestinal haemorrhage is probably the next most common mode of death in the acute period. This occurs in about 5% of severe spinal injuries, particularly when other injuries are associated, or acute surgery is performed.

*Cardio-respiratory arrest*   Another fairly common cause of death is sudden cardio-respiratory arrest, often from causes

81

unknown. It may be from vasovagal inhibition, or secondary to a respiratory arrest from a ventilation problem.

*Pulmonary embolus*   Massive pulmonary embolus may be the cause of death, secondary to undiagnosed deep vein thrombosis, usually in the leg.

## Delayed Causes of Death

*Renal failure*   Chronic death is defined as death occurring more than 2 months after the onset of spinal paralysis. The commonest cause of death is from renal failure secondary to hydronephrosis, pyelonephritis, renal calculi, renal amyloidosis, or a combination of these.

In most series, renal deaths now account for less than 50% of delayed causes of death.

*Chest complications*   Another delayed cause of death is from chest complications, usually following upper respiratory tract infections in quadriplegics. Here the same cycle of events occurs as in the acute stage, with pulmonary collapse and consolidation secondary to accumulation of bronchial secretions, and superimposed broncho or lobar pneumonia. Death from chest complications may occur within 24 hours of onset of symptoms.

*Pressure sores*   Multiple pressure sores with involvement of bone and joint, and chronic sepsis can be the cause of death in a patient in as short a period as 6 weeks.

*Suicide*   In patients with such a severe disability as that of a spinal patient, it would be expected that suicide would be a ranking cause of death. This is not so. Suicide in spinal patients is no higher than in the normal population. When suicide is attempted, it may be actively with drugs of self-mutilation, or passively by self-neglect leading to all the complications of paraplegia.

82

# SOCIAL ASPECTS OF REHABILITATION

There are several problem areas encountered in dealing with the spinal patient which, although not medical, must be considered. These problems touch upon other specialised fields, so they will only be briefly outlined.

## Litigation

Every effort must be made to ensure that the patient is aware of his legal position, and that a solicitor or insurance company is properly informed of the case. These problems are a tremendous source of worry to the patient and may adversely influence his recovery.

### Family

Immediate family members must be accurately and honestly informed of the patient's injury and prognosis as soon as possible. Support and advice by the social worker is essential. This care must be on a continuing basis, not only while the patient is in hospital, but also during his resettlement in the community after discharge. Such support may take the form of assisting the family in making arrangements for child care when the mother is injured. The social worker may be pressed into service as a marital counsellor upon occasions.

### Finances

Financial aid might have to be sought for a family that has an injured wage earner, and that has no financial resources. This aid may have to continue until the patient is re-employed or retrained. Social workers are excellent in dealing with the complexities of government finances, pension plans, disability allowances and so forth.

## Employment

After such a severe injury, the patient may have to change jobs or be retrained for another job. He may have to work in a sheltered workshop. This must be planned before discharge from hospital, so the patient knows what he will be doing and where, when he is ready for home. To be able to return to the family as a wage earner is of great psychological (and financial) importance to the spinal patient. Further, it completes the aim of rehabilitation—that of getting the patient back into the community and back to work.

## Home

Advice will be necessary in most cases for adaptation of the home for wheelchair living. Ramps, wide doorways, accessible toilets, appropriate bathing facilities, kitchen modifications for the housewife are just some of the considerations. This can be handled by qualified people making home visits, and then making recommendations to the family concerned.

## Tertiary Placement

Sometimes, returning the patient to the home is not possible, either because of the severity of his handicap, or because there is nobody who can take care of him in the home. Alternatives must be found, and usually take the form of nursing homes. These are less than satisfactory, as the patient ends up being institutionalised in a place filled with chronically ill people much older than himself. It is difficult for him to get out to socialise—so he is stuck there. The quality of medical care for the spinal patient is below standard in most instances. Hopefully, specialised spinal patient hostels are on the not-too-distant horizon, wherein the severely handicapped and homeless spinal patient can be cared for without being totally institutionalised, thus maintaining a quality of life which will make it all worthwhile to him.

# Selected Bibliography

## Journals

*Functional Anatomy of the Spinal Column*

Munro, D., 'Factors Governing the Stability of the Spine', *Paraplegia*, **3**, 219 (1965)

Romanes, G. T., 'The Arterial Supply of the Human Spinal Cord', *Paraplegia*, **2**, 199 (1964)

*Spinal Column Injuries*

Bedbrook, G. M., 'Some Pertinent Observations on the Pathology of Traumatic Spinal Paralysis', *Paraplegia*, **1**, 215 (1963)

Bedbrook, G. M., 'Pathological Principles in the Initial Treatment of Traumatic Spinal Cord Damage', *Paraplegia*, **3**, 65 (1965)

Burke, D. C., 'Spinal Cord Trauma in Children', *Paraplegia*, **9**, 297 (1971)

Burke, D. C., 'Hyperextension Injuries of the Spine', *J.B.J.S.*, **53B**, 3 (1971)

Burke, D. C., 'Traumatic Spinal Paralysis in Children', *Paraplegia*, **11**, 268–276 (1974)

Burke, D. C. and Berryman, D., 'The Place of Closed Manipulation in the Management of Flexion-Rotation Dislocations of the Cervical Spine', *J.B.J.S.*, **53B**, 165 (1971)

Cheshire, D. J. E., 'The Complete and Centralised Treatment of Paraplegia', *Paraplegia*, **6**, 59 (1959)

Cheshire, D. J. E., 'The Stability of the Cervical Spine Following Conservative Treatment of Fractures and Fracture-Dislocations', *Paraplegia*, **7**, 193 (1969)

Evans, D. K., 'Reduction of Cervical Dislocations', *J.B.J.S.*, **43B**, 552 (1961)

Geisler, W. D., Wynn-Jones, M. and Jousse, A., 'Early Management of the Patient with Trauma to the Spinal Cord', *Med. Services Journal of Canada*, **22**, 698 (1966)

Guttman, L., 'The Treatment and Rehabilitation of Patients

with Injuries of the Spinal Cord', in Cope, Z., *History of World War II,* United Kingdom Medical Services (1953)

Guttman, L., 'Spinal Deformities in Traumatic Paraplegics and Tetraplegics Following Spinal Procedures', *Paraplegia,* 7, 38 (1969)

Hardy, A. G., 'The Treatment of Paraplegia due to Fracture-Dislocations of the Dorso-lumbar Spine', *Paraplegia,* 3, 112 (1965)

Holdsworth, F. W., 'Fractures, Dislocations and Fracture-Dislocations of the Spine', *J.B.J.S.,* 45B, 6 (1963)

Jousse, A. T., 'The Management of Paraplegia', *Manitoba Medical Review,* 43, 7 (1963)

Lipschitz, R. and Block, J., 'Stab Wounds of the Spinal Cord', *Lancet,* 2, 169 (1962)

Morgan, T. H., Wharton, G. W. and Austin, G. N., 'The Results of Laminectomy in Patients with Incomplete Spinal Cord Injuries', *Paraplegia,* 9, 14 (1971)

*Spinal Cord Injuries*

Schneider, R. C., 'The Syndrome of Acute Anterior Spinal Cord Injury', *Journal Neuro.,* 11, 546 (1954); *Journal Neuro.,* 12, 95 (1955)

Schneider, R. C. and Kahn, E. A., 'Chronic Neurological Sequelae of Acute Trauma to the Spinal Cord', *J.B.J.S.,* 38A, 985 (1952)

*Management of the Acute Spinal Patient*

Cheshire, D. J. E. and Coats, D. A., 'Respiratory and Metabolic Management in Acute Tetraplegia', *Paraplegia,* 4, 8 (1966)

Johnson, R. H., 'Temperature Regulation in Paraplegia', *Paraplegia,* 9, 137 (1971)

Perret, G. and Solomon, A., 'Gastrointestinal Haemorrhage and Cervical Cord Lesions', Proceedings of 17th Veterans Administrat. Spinal Cord Injury Conference, N.Y. (1969)

*Neurogenic Bladder*

Burr, R. G., 'Urinary Calcium, Magnesium, Crystals and Stones in Paraplegia', *Paraplegia,* 10, 56 (1972)

Cosbie-Ross, J., 'Diversion of the Urine in Paraplegia', *Paraplegia*, **4**, 209 (1967)

Damanski, M., 'Stone Disease in Paraplegia', *Paraplegia*, **1**, 148 (1963)

Gibbon, N. O. K., Ross, J. C. and Silver, J. R., 'Changes in the Upper Urinary Tract Following Various Types of Initial Treatment', *Paraplegia*, **7**, 63 (1969)

Guttman, L. and Frankel, H., 'The Value of Intermittent Catheterisation in the Early Management of Traumatic Paraplegia and Tetraplegia', *Paraplegia*, **4**, 63 (1966)

Hardy, A. G., 'Complications of the Indwelling Urethral Catheter', *Paraplegia*, **6**, 5 (1968)

Lindan, R., 'The Prevention of Ascending Catheter-induced Infection of the Urinary Tract', *J. Chron. Dis.*, 321 (1969)

Pearman, J. W., 'Prevention of Urinary Tract Infection Following Spinal Cord Injury', *Paraplegia*, **9**, 95 (1971)

Retief, P. J. M. and Key, A. G., 'Urinary Diversion in Paraplegia', *Paraplegia*, **4**, 225 (1967)

Smith, P. H., Cook, J. B. and Rhind, J. R., 'Manual Expression of the Bladder Following Spinal Injury', *Paraplegia*, **9**, 213 (1972)

*Sexual Function*

Cole, T. M., Chilgren, R. and Rosenberg, P., 'A New Programme of Sex Education and Counselling for Spinal Cord Injured Adults and Health Care Professionals, *Paraplegia*, **11**, 111–124 (1973)

Comarr, A. E., 'Sexual Concepts in Traumatic Cord and Cauda Equina Lesions', *J. Urol.*, **106**, 375 (1971)

Guttman, L., 'The Married Life of Paraplegics and Tetra-plegics', *Paraplegia*, **2**, 182 (1964)

Robertson, D. N. S., 'Pregnancy and Labour in the Paraplegic', *Paraplegia*, **10**, 209 (1972)

Talbot, H. S., 'Psycho-social Aspects of Sexuality in Spinal Cord Injury Patients', *Paraplegia*, **9**, 37 (1971)

Tarabulcy, E., 'Sexual Function in the Normal and in Paraplegia', *Paraplegia*, **10**, 201 (1972)

*Ascending Myelopathy*

Barnett, H. J. M., Botterell, E. H., Jousse, A. T. and Wynn-Jones, M., 'Progressive Myelopathy as a Sequela to Traumatic Paraplegia', *Med. Services Journal Canada*, **22**, 7 (1966)

Jousse, A. *et al.*, 'Post Traumatic Syringomyelia', *Paraplegia*, **9**, 33 (1971)


*Chronic Pain*

Botterell, E. H., Callaghan, J. G. and Jousse, A. T., 'Pain in Paraplegia—Clinical Management and Surgical Treatment', *Proc. Royal Soc. Med.*, **47**, 4 (1954)

Burke, D. C., 'Pain in Paraplegia', *Paraplegia*, **10**, 297 (1973)


*Para-articular Heterotopic Ossification*

Rossier, A., 'Current Facts on Para-Osteo-Arthropathy (P.O.A.)', *Paraplegia*, **11**, 36 (1973)

Wharton, G. W. and Morgan, T. H., 'Ankylosis in the Paralysed Patient', *J.B.J.S.*, **52A**, 105 (1970)


*Osteoporosis and Pathological Fractures*

Benassy, J., 'Associated Fractures of the Limbs in Traumatic Paraplegia and Tetraplegia', *Paraplegia*, **5**, 209 (1968)


*Aims in Rehabilitation*

Cheshire, D. J. E., 'A Classification of the Functional End Results of Injury to the Cervical Spinal Cord', *Paraplegia*, **8**, 70 (1970)

Maling, R., 'Electronic Controls for the Tetraplegic (P.O.S.S.U.M.)', *Paraplegia*, **1**, 78 and 161 (1963)

Stauffer, E. S. and Nickel, V. L., 'Control Systems for Upper Extremity Function in Traumatic Quadriplegia', *Paraplegia*, **10**, 3 (1972)

Trigiano, L. L., 'Physical Rehabilitation of Quadriplegic Patients', *Arch. Phys. Med.*, **51**, 592 (1972)

*Mortality*
Breithaupt, D. J., Jousse, A. T. and Wynn-Jones, M., 'Late Causes of Death and Life Expectancy in Paraplegia', *C.M.A.J.*, **85**, 73 (1961)
Price, M., 'Causes of Death in 227 Patients with Traumatic Spinal Cord Injury Over a Period of Nine Years', *Paraplegia,* **11,** 217–220 (1974)
Nyquist, H. and Bors, E., 'Mortality and Survival in Traumatic Myelopathy', *Paraplegia,* **5,** 22 (1967)
Tribe, C. R., 'Causes of Death in the Early and Late Stages of Paraplegia', *Paraplegia,* **1,** 19 (1963)

*Social Aspects of Rehabilitation*
Barrie, D., 'Non-medical Management of Spinal Cord Injury', *Paraplegia,* **11,** 96 (1973)
Harris, P., Patel, S. S., Greer, W. and Naughton, J. A. L., 'Psychological and Social Reactions to Acute Spinal Paralysis', *Paraplegia,* **11,** 132–136 (1973)

## Reference Texts

Austin, G., *The Spinal Cord,* C. C. Thomas, Springfield (1961)
Bors, E. and Comarr, A. E., *Neurological Urology,* S. Karger, Basel (1971)
Breakman, R. (Editor), *Handbook of Clinical Neurology, Vols 24/25, Injuries of the Spinal Cord and Column,* North Holland, Amsterdam, to be published
Guttman, L., *Spinal Cord Injuries—Comprehensive Management and Research,* Blackwell (1973)
Harris, P. (Editor), *Spinal Injuries—A Symposium,* Royal College of Surgeons, Edinburgh (1963)
Hughes, J. T., *Pathology of the Spinal Cord,* Lloyd-Luke, London (1966)
Pearman, J. W. and England, E., *The Urological Management of the Patient Following Spinal Injury,* C. C. Thomas, Springfield (1972)
Rossier, A., *Rehabilitation of the Spinal Cord Patient,*

Documenta Geigy Acta Clinica, Basel (1973)

Ruge, D., *Spinal Cord Injury,* C. C. Thomas, Springfield (1969)

Sutton, N., *Injuries of the Spinal Cord,* Butterworths, London (1973)